Easy One Pot

without the calories

Justine Pattison

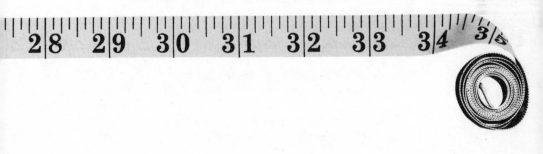

SEVEN DIALS

First published in Great Britain in 2015 by Orion Publishing Group
This reissued edition published in 2020 by Seven Dials
an imprint of The Orion Publishing Group Ltd
Carmelite House, 50 Victoria Embankment
London EC4Y 0DZ

An Hachette UK Company

1 3 5 7 9 10 8 6 4 2

Text © Justine Pattison 2015
Design and layout © Orion 2015
Photography by Cristian Barnett

A CIP catalogue record for this book is
available from the British Library.

ISBN (Trade paperback) 978 1 8418 8445 5
ISBN (eBook) 978 1 4091 5480 8

Printed and bound in Great Britain by Clays Ltd, Elcograf, S.p.A

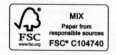

www.orionbooks.co.uk

For Damon

Also in the *Without the Calories* series

Takeway Favourites Without the Calories

Quick and Easy Without the Calories

Slow Cooker Without the Calories

Pasta and Rice Without the Calories

Cakes, Cookies and Bread Without the Calories

Comfort Food Without the Calories

Also by Justine Pattison

Fill Your Freezer

The Healthy Gut Handbook

Contents

Contents

introduction

MY STORY

I struggled with my weight for years. After being a skinny child and teenager, I piled on the weight during my last years of school and went into my twenties feeling fat and frumpy. A career as a cookery writer and food stylist has helped me understand good food but because my kitchen is always overflowing with great things to eat, temptation is never far away. My weight yo-yoed for twenty years and at my heaviest I weighed more than 15 stone.

A few years ago, I worked on the hit TV series *You Are What You Eat* – I put together those groaning tables of bad food. I also had the chance to work with the contributors on the show, guiding them through the dieting process and helping them discover a whole new way of eating and cooking. Having been overweight myself, I became passionate about helping people lose weight.

Since then, I've worked as a food consultant on many of the weight-loss shows you've seen on TV, and written diet plans and recipes for best-selling books, newspapers and magazines. I'm thrilled that thousands of people have successfully followed my way of cooking and lost weight.

This book, and the others in the *Without the Calories* series, are ideal for anyone who wants to lose weight while leading a normal life. Cooking my way will help you sustain a happy, healthy weight loss. That's what it's all about: you don't have to be stick thin, but you deserve to feel good about yourself. My Without the Calories recipes will help you reach your goal.

ABOUT THIS BOOK

When you are busy, finding time to shop and cook can be tough – and it's not just the preparation – by the time you've finished your meal, there could be a stack of washing-up waiting to be done too.

In this book, I've minimised the work and cleaning up needed to create a host of easy, delicious and complete low-calorie meals. Most recipes only require one dish – whether it's a saucepan, wok, casserole or serving bowl. Sometimes a recipe will require a bowl or plate for mixing ingredients or measuring, for a dressing or sauce for instance, but I've kept the call for additional equipment as low as possible.

I've reworked the ingredients and used crafty cooking methods to reduce the calories while ensuring that every dish remains as delicious as possible. There are no complicated methods, just simple food cooked without fuss.

I'm not going to make rash promises about how many pounds you will shed, but I do know that when it comes to losing weight, finding foods that give you pleasure and fit into your lifestyle are the key to success. When you eat well without obsessing over rapid weight loss, it's easier to relax and lose what you need to comfortably – and safely.

To help everyone enjoy these reinvented dishes, I've used easy-to-find ingredients and given clear, simple cooking instructions. There's also freezer information included where approproate, so you know which dishes you can store safely for another day.

If you're already following a diet plan, you'll find additional nutritional information at the back of the book that'll help you work my recipes into your week. And, if you're stuck for inspiration and have a few pounds to lose, try my 123 Plan. It couldn't be easier.

USING THE 123 PLAN

It works on the basis of three meals a day, with each belonging to a different calorie group listed below: ONE, TWO or THREE. You want your daily intake to be between 900 and 1,200 calories. Make sure to go to page 191 for *essential extras* if you're under this calorie amount and for a list of 'free' vegetables you should include with your meals. Make sure to join the community at justinepattison.com and check out the other books in the *Without the Calories* series.

ONE
up to 300 calories

TWO
300–400 calories

THREE
400–560 calories

YOUR ESSENTIAL EXTRAS

These extra 300 calories can be made up of accompaniments, such as potatoes, rice and pasta, as well as snacks or treats; there are suggestions and serving sizes on page 191. You'll also find recipes that contain under 200 calories per portion, which can be included as part of your essential extras. As long as your extras don't exceed 300 calories a day, you'll be on track.

DON'T RUSH IT

Weight tends to be gained over time, and losing it gradually will make the process easier and help give your body, especially your skin, time to adapt. You're more likely to get into positive, enjoyable long-term cooking and eating habits this way too.

WHAT IS A CALORIE?

Put simply, a calorie is a unit of energy contained within food and drink which our bodies burn as fuel. Different foods contain varying amounts of calories and if more calories are consumed than the body needs, the excess will be stored as fat. To lose weight, we need to eat less or use more energy by increasing our activity – and ideally both!

I've provided the calorie content of a single serving of each dish. In my experience, most people will lose at least 2lb a week by consuming around 1,200–1,500 calories a day, but it's always best to check with your GP before you start a new regime. Everyone is different and, especially if you have several stones to lose, you'll need some personalised advice. The calories contained in each recipe have been calculated as accurately as possible, but could vary a little depending on your ingredients. If you have a couple of days of eating more than 1,400 calories, try to eat closer to 1,100 for the next few days. Over a week, things will even out.

My recipes strike a balance between eating and cooking well and reducing calories, and I've tried them all as part of my own way of enjoying food without putting on excess weight. Even if you don't need to lose weight, I hope you enjoy cooking from my books simply because you like the recipes.

SECRETS OF SUCCESS

The serving sizes that I've recommended form the basis of the nutritional information on page 195, and if you eat any more, you may find losing weight takes longer. If you're cooking for anyone who doesn't need to watch their calorie intake, you can increase their servings, but bear in mind that too much sugar isn't good for anyone.

The right portion size also holds the key to maintaining your weight loss. Use this opportunity to get used to smaller servings. Work out exactly how much food your body needs to maintain the shape that makes you feel great. That way, even when counting calories feels like a distant memory, you'll remain in control of your eating habits.

Stick to lean protein (which will help you feel fuller for longer) and vegetables and avoid high-fat, high-sugar snacks and confectionery. Be aware that alcohol is packed with empty calories and could weaken your resolve. Starchy carbs such as pasta, rice, potatoes and bread are kept to a minimum because I've found that, combined with eating lots of veg and good protein, this leads to more sustainable weight loss. There's no need to avoid dairy products such as cheese and cream, although they tend to be high in fat and calories. You can swap the high-fat versions for reduced-fat ones, or use less.

Ditch heavily processed foods and you will feel so much better. Switching to more natural ingredients will help your body work with you.

Most recipes in the *Without the Calories* series form the main part of each meal, so there's room to have your plate half-filled with freshly cooked vegetables or a colourful, crunchy salad. This will help fill you up, and boost your intake of vitamins and minerals.

Make sure you drink enough fluids, especially water – around 2 litres is ideal. Staying hydrated will help you lose weight more comfortably, and it's important when you exercise too.

IN THE KITCHEN

Pick up some electronic kitchen scales and a set of measuring spoons if you don't already have them. Both will probably cost less than a takeaway meal for two, and will help ensure good results.

Invest, if you can, in a large, deep non-stick frying pan, a medium non-stick saucepan and a large saucepan for pasta (so it can bubble freely). The non-stick coating means that you will need less oil to cook, and a frying pan with a wide base and deep sides can double as a wok. Non-stick baking parchment will prevent sticking and means you can use less oil. Look at the oven temperatures carefully. All the recipes in this book have been tested using a fan oven setting, which is always best for baking.

I use oil and butter sparingly, and use a mild olive oil spray for frying. I also keep a jam jar containing a little sunflower oil and a heatproof pastry brush to hand for greasing pans lightly before baking and frying.

STICK WITH IT

Shifting your eating habits and trying to lose weight is not easy, especially if you have been eating the same way for many years. But it isn't too late. You may never have the perfect body, but you can have one that, fuelled by really good food, makes you feel happy and healthy. For more information, tips and ideas, make sure you visit visit justinepattison.com.

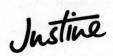

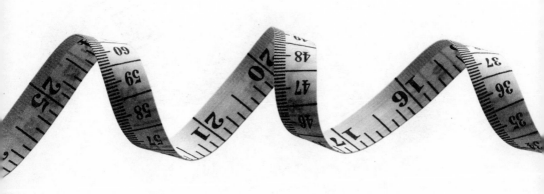

| baking tray

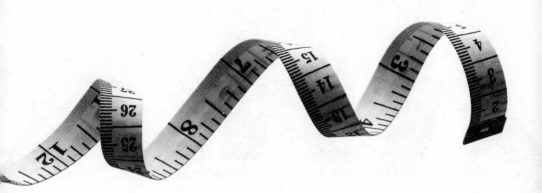

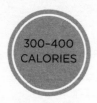

353
CALORIES
PER SERVING

SERVES 4

PREP: 10 MINUTES

COOK: 40 MINUTES

INGREDIENTS

oil, for spraying or brushing

500g medium potatoes (ideally Maris
   Piper), peeled and cut into roughly
   2.5cm chunks

4 boneless, skinless chicken breasts
   (each about 175g)

4 thin slices of Emmental or Gruyère cheese
   (each slice about 25g)

4 thin slices of prosciutto or serrano ham

250g bunch slender asparagus spears,
   trimmed and halved

flaked sea salt

ground black pepper

Tip: Use thin cheese slices from a resealable pack for stuffing the
chicken. Freeze any leftover cheese for up to 1 month.

quick cheesy chicken and ham

Cheese-filled chicken breasts wrapped in prosciutto and roasted with potatoes and asparagus. What's not to like?

Preheat the oven to 200°C/Fan 180°C/Gas 6. Spray or brush a large baking tray with oil, add the potatoes, spray with more oil and season with salt and pepper. Roast for 15 minutes.

While the potatoes are cooking, place one of the chicken breasts on a board with the smooth side underneath. Using a sharp knife, carefully cut horizontally through the breast from the curved side almost all the way through to the other side and open it out like a book. You may need to cut a little way, then gently flip the breast open and carry on gently cutting through the meat so it opens easily without tearing.

Place a slice of cheese over the open chicken breast and fold the chicken back over to completely enclose the cheese. Repeat with the other chicken breasts. Wrap each chicken breast in a slice of ham, to seal the cheese inside, season generously with salt and pepper and set aside.

Take the baking tray out of the oven and turn the potatoes. Nestle the chicken breasts among the potatoes, spray with a little oil and roast for 15 more minutes.

Take the baking tray out of the oven once more and dot the asparagus spears among the chicken and vegetables. Return to the oven for a further 10–12 minutes, or until the chicken is cooked through and the asparagus is just tender. Serve on warmed plates.

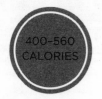

461

CALORIES
PER SERVING

SERVES 4

PREP: 15 MINUTES

COOK: 1–1¼ HOURS

INGREDIENTS

1 chicken (about 1.2kg)

330ml can Diet Coke or diet lemonade

800g medium potatoes (ideally Maris
    Piper), peeled and quartered into
    roughly 4cm chunks

oil, for spraying or brushing

2 bushy thyme sprigs, leaves stripped
    off (optional)

1–2 rosemary sprigs, leaves stripped off
    (optional)

flaked sea salt

ground black pepper

large mixed salad, to serve

chipotle mayo (see page 7), to serve

soda can roast chicken

This is a fab way of roasting a chicken and it guarantees delicious roasted potatoes. If you stand the chicken on a can of fizzy Coke or lemonade, it stays moist, cooks more quickly and saves space in the roasting tin. If you have the chicken with skin the calories will increase to 539 per serving.

Preheat the oven to 200°C/Fan 180°C/Gas 6. Rearrange the shelves so you just have one shelf on the bottom rung, leaving space for the chicken to stand upright.

Untruss the chicken by removing the string. Season all over with salt and pepper. Open the can of Coke or lemonade and drink or pour away half of it. There should be enough left to hold the chicken steady when it sits on top of the can.

Put the potatoes in a large roasting tin and spray or brush with oil. Season well with salt and pepper and make a small gap in the centre. Set the can in the gap and ease the chicken on top of it.

Roast the chicken for 30 minutes, then take the roasting tin out of the oven very carefully and turn all the potatoes. Sprinkle with thyme and rosemary leaves, if using. Return to the oven for a further 30–45 minutes or until the chicken is thoroughly cooked and the potatoes are golden.

Remove the roasting tin from the oven and very carefully lift the chicken off the can – you may need someone to hold the can with an oven glove while you lift the chicken. Discard the liquid inside the can. Put the chicken on a board and carve. Divide the chicken and potatoes between four warmed plates. Serve with a large salad and the chipotle mayo see page 7.

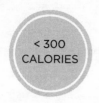

65

CALORIES
PER SERVING

SERVES 4

PREP: 5 MINUTES

INGREDIENTS

75g reduced-fat mayonnaise

50g fat-free fromage frais

2 tsp chipotle paste (from a jar)

1 tsp fresh lemon juice

1 garlic clove, crushed or finely grated

smoked paprika (optional)

flaked sea salt

ground black pepper

Tip: Chipotle paste is made from smoked jalapeño peppers. It's available in larger supermarkets but you can substitute with harissa paste, which will give a different but just as delicious flavour, or leave it out altogether to make a garlic mayo. If you can't get hold of fat-free fromage frais, use natural yoghurt instead, the calories will be slightly different but not enough to worry about.

chipotle mayo

This really is a very simple, but effective sauce. The chipotle paste will last in the fridge for weeks and can be used to marinade meat or fish and works really well if you want to make some spicy sweet potato wedges. To make the chipotle mayo, all you need to do is mix all of the ingredients together and serve immediately. You can dial the heat up or down depending on how much paste you add, but 2 teaspoons will give you a moderate heat.

Put the mayonnaise, fromage frais, chipotle paste, lemon juice and garlic in a small bowl and mix well. Leave to stand for a few minutes to allow the flavours to mingle.

Add a little salt and pepper to taste and sprinkle with a little smoked paprika if you like.

Serve with the soda can roast chicken on page 5, any other grilled or roasted meat of fish, or as a dip with vegetable sticks.

If the chipotle mayo doesn't get eaten all at once with the chicken, any leftover can be covered and kept in the fridge for up to 2 days. Stir well before using.

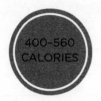

463

CALORIES
PER SERVING

SERVES 4

PREP: 20 MINUTES

COOK: 1 HOUR 10 MINUTES

INGREDIENTS

500g medium potatoes (ideally Maris Piper), peeled and cut into roughly 4cm chunks

4 medium carrots (each about 100g), peeled and cut into 5cm long batons

2 medium parsnips (each about 150g), peeled and cut into 5cm long batons

oil, for spraying or brushing

40g dried sage and onion stuffing mix

8 boneless, skinless chicken thighs (about 675g), trimmed of visible fat

4 lean smoked back bacon rashers (about 125g), trimmed of visible fat and cut into 3cm slices

150g thin long-stemmed broccoli, trimmed and rinsed in cold water

2 tbsp Marsala or Madeira

250ml chicken stock (made with ½ chicken cube)

1 tbsp redcurrant jelly

flaked sea salt

ground black pepper

all-in-one roast chicken dinner

A brilliant way to feed the family with hardly any washing-up! The chicken pieces, all the vegetables and even the gravy is cooked in one tin. Use a roasting tin or baking tray with a good thick base as it will need to go on the hob to make the gravy. If your tray is a little flimsy, deglaze the pan with the stock to collect all the juicy bits, then make the gravy in a small saucepan. Sprinkling the chicken with stuffing mix adds a lovely herb flavour and a bit of crunch.

Preheat the oven to 200°C/Fan 180°C/Gas 6. Put the potatoes, carrots and parsnips in a large roasting tin or baking tray and spray or brush generously with the oil. Season with salt and pepper and roast for 25 minutes.

Put the stuffing mix in a sturdy freezer bag. Take the tin of vegetables out of the oven and turn them over.

Drop the chicken thighs one at a time into the bag with the stuffing mix and turn to coat. Place the thighs among the vegetables, arranging them into nice neat shapes. Spray or brush with more oil and bake for a further 25 minutes.

Take the roasting tin out of the oven and add the bacon slices and broccoli, nestling them among the chicken pieces and root vegetables. Spray with a little more oil. Return to the oven for a further 15 minutes or until the chicken is cooked through and lightly browned, and the vegetables are tender.

Transfer the contents of the roasting tin to a warmed platter or serving dish. Place the roasting tin on the hob and pour over the Marsala or Madeira and the stock. Add the redcurrant jelly and bring to a simmer. Cook for 2–3 minutes or until the liquid has reduced by half, stirring to scrape up the juicy bits from the

all-in-one roast
chicken dinner (continued)

bottom of the pan. Season to taste with salt and pepper then strain into a small warmed jug. Serve with the chicken and vegetables.

Tips: Use red or white wine instead of the Marsala for the gravy if you like, and add ½ teaspoon caster sugar.

Use kitchen scissors to remove the visible fat from the chicken.

Making lasting changes to your diet and lifestyle is a big deal and no-one achieves their aims 100% of the time. This book is designed to make it as easy as possible, but if you do end up eating more than you intended, don't beat yourself up about it. Start again with the next meal and aim to balance things out over the course of the week.

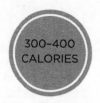

300–400
CALORIES

381
CALORIES
PER SERVING

SERVES 4

PREP: 15 MINUTES

COOK: 40 MINUTES

INGREDIENTS

1 tsp smoked paprika

1 tsp ground black pepper, plus extra
to season

½ tsp fine sea salt, plus extra to season

8 boneless, skinless chicken thighs (about
675g), trimmed of visible fat

2 x 200g potatoes (ideally a floury variety
such as King Edward or Maris Piper),
washed, patted dry and each cut into
10–12 long wedges

oil, for spraying or brushing

2 sweetcorn cobs (each about 250g)

1 tbsp cold water

10g butter

large mixed salad, to serve

For the barbecue sauce

3 tbsp tomato ketchup

1½ tbsp clear honey

1 tbsp Worcestershire sauce

barbecue-style chicken with potato wedges and corn

This is a dish that all the family will enjoy. The chicken pieces are deliciously sticky and sweet and the potatoes and corn can be conveniently baked in the oven alongside them. If you do have any chicken left over, it's great served with salad for lunch the next day.

Preheat the oven to 200°C/Fan 180°C/Gas 6. Line the base and sides of a large baking tray with a piece of foil (this will stop the sauce sticking and making the tray difficult to clean).

Put the paprika, pepper and salt in a large freezer bag. Carefully slash each chicken thigh 2–3 times with a sharp knife. Add the chicken to the bag with the seasoning and toss well until it is lightly coated. Place the chicken on the lined tray, arranging the thighs into nice neat shapes.

Place the potato wedges at one end of the same tray as the chicken and spray or brush with oil. Season with salt and pepper.

Cut the two sweetcorn cobs in half widthways and place them on a large square of foil. Bring up the sides and pour the cold water over the cobs. Add the butter and fold over the top tightly to make a sealed parcel.

Place the chicken and potatoes on the top shelf of the oven and put the foil parcel containing the sweetcorn on the shelf beneath. Bake for 30 minutes.

To make the barbecue sauce, mix the ingredients together in a bowl. Take the baking tray out of the oven, turn the potatoes and spoon the sauce liberally over the chicken. Return to the oven and cook for a further 10 minutes. Serve the chicken, wedges and corn with a large mixed salad.

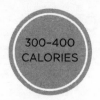

361
CALORIES
PER SERVING

SERVES 4

PREP: 15 MINUTES

COOK: 50-65 MINUTES

INGREDIENTS

2 medium red onions, each cut into 8 wedges

500g potatoes (ideally Maris Piper), peeled and cut into roughly 3cm chunks

4 large tomatoes, quartered

oil, for spraying

8 boneless, skinless chicken thighs (about 675g), trimmed of visible fat

1 large red pepper, deseeded and cut into roughly 3cm chunks

1 large yellow pepper, deseeded and cut into roughly 3cm chunks

½ tsp sweet smoked paprika

½ tsp dried oregano

1 large lemon, halved lengthways

flaked sea salt

ground black pepper

chopped flat-leaf parsley, to garnish (optional)

lemony chicken tray bake

A light and summery dish of tender chicken thighs baked with lots of colourful vegetables and lemony roast potatoes. A little olive oil can be drizzled over the top, but you'll need to add around 80 calories for each tablespoon. Serve with a lightly dressed green salad, if you like.

Preheat the oven to 200°C/Fan 180°C/Gas 6. Put the onions, potatoes and tomatoes in a large roasting tin or scatter them over a large baking tray and season with salt and lots of freshly ground black pepper. Spray with oil and toss together lightly. Roast for 20 minutes.

While the vegetables are roasting, put the chicken thighs on a board. Carefully slash each thigh 2–3 times with a knife.

Take the roasting tin or baking tray out of the oven, add the pepper chunks and turn the vegetables a couple of times. Place the chicken in the tin or tray and season all over with black pepper. Mix the paprika and oregano together and sprinkle over the top. Thickly slice one half of the lemon and add to the tin. Squeeze the juice from the other half over the chicken and vegetables.

Return to the oven for a further 30–45 minutes, or until the vegetables are tender and lightly charred and the chicken is thoroughly cooked. Plate the chicken and vegetables and spoon over the lemony tomato cooking juices. Garnish with chopped parsley, if you like.

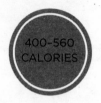

556
CALORIES
PER SERVING

SERVES 6

PREP: 20 MINUTES

**COOK: 2½ HOURS,
PLUS RESTING TIME**

INGREDIENTS

1.5kg whole leg of lamb

800g medium potatoes (ideally
  Maris Piper)

500g medium-large carrots

500g medium-large parsnips

oil, for spraying or brushing

300g fine green beans, trimmed

flaked sea salt

ground black pepper

For the gravy

2 tbsp plain flour

100ml red wine

500ml hot lamb stock (made with
  1 lamb cube)

1 tbsp redcurrant jelly

no-fuss roast lamb

I thought a lot about this recipe and was originally planning something quite fancy. In the end, however, I opted for the sort of meal my family like to eat regularly. There isn't anything unusual about this simple combination of ingredients, but it's easy to knock together and great for lunch on a busy Sunday.

Preheat the oven to 200°C/Fan 180°C/Gas 6. Place the lamb in a large, sturdy roasting tin and season well with salt and pepper. Roast for 1¼ hours.

While the lamb is roasting, prepare all the vegetables. Peel and quarter the potatoes and peel the carrots and parsnips and cut them into short batons, each about 4cm long and 1.5cm wide. Keeping them a similar size will help them cook more evenly and because they are small, they will cook quickly, too.

Take the lamb out of the oven and transfer it to a board. Place the vegetables into the tin and spray or brush with oil. Season with salt and pepper and toss well together. Place the lamb on top of the vegetables and return to the oven for a further hour.

Remove the tin from the oven and transfer the lamb to a board again. Loosely cover with foil and a couple of folded tea towels. Add the green beans to the roasting tin and turn the root vegetables and beans. Return to the oven for 10 minutes or until the beans are just tender.

Transfer the vegetables to a warmed serving dish and place the roasting tin on the hob. To make the gravy, stir the flour into the meat juices with a wooden spoon, then slowly add the stock, stirring well between each addition. Add the wine and redcurrant jelly and bring to the boil. Cook for 1 minute. If your gravy is still a little lumpy, whisk hard with a metal whisk until smooth. Season with salt and pepper and strain through a fine

no-fuss roast lamb
(continued)

sieve into a warmed jug. Carve the lamb, discarding as much fat as possible, add any resting juices to the gravy and serve with fresh mint sauce (see page 21), the vegetables and gravy for pouring.

Tip: Use a roasting tin or baking tray with a thick base as it will need to go on the hob to make the gravy. If your tray is a little flimsy, deglaze the pan with the stock to collect all the juicy bits, then make the gravy in a small saucepan.

Returning to your favourite dishes is a comforting ritual, which is why this book is full of healthier takes on the classics. But mixing things up keeps any eating plan interesting, so try to cook something new occasionally too. Tweaking the spices or citrus in a marinade can also make a difference without dramatically altering the calories.

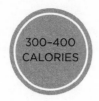

308
CALORIES
PER SERVING

SERVES 2

PREP: 15 MINUTES

COOK: 40 MINUTES

INGREDIENTS

1 rack of lamb, extra trimmed (about 300g)

oil, for spraying or brushing

150g baby carrots, trimmed and halved
   if large

300g baby new potatoes, halved

200g baby courgettes, trimmed

flaked sea salt

ground black pepper

For the fresh mint sauce

15g bunch of fresh mint, leaves stripped
   from stalks and finely chopped

1 tbsp caster sugar

1 tbsp white wine vinegar

4 tbsp just-boiled water

lamb with spring vegetables and mint

Look out for extra-trimmed racks of lamb for this recipe as all the hard work will have been done for you. They usually have 6 or 7 little rib bones that you can carve between to serve. Rack of lamb is fairly pricey, so keep this lovely dish for a special occasion.

Preheat the oven to 200°C/Fan 180°C/Gas 6. Season the lamb all over with a little salt and plenty of freshly ground black pepper. Brush or spray a sturdy, medium baking tray with oil and place over a medium-high heat.

Once the tin is hot but not smoking, carefully place the rack in the pan. Cook for 3½–4 minutes, turning the rack after each minute with tongs to ensure that every side of the lamb is lightly browned. Set aside on a board.

Add the carrots and potatoes to the roasting tin and spray or brush with oil. Season with salt and lots of freshly ground black pepper. Roast in the oven for 15 minutes.

Meanwhile, make the mint sauce. Put the chopped mint leaves in a small bowl and stir in the sugar and vinegar. Add 4 tablespoons of just-boiled water and stir well. Leave to cool.

Take the carrots and potatoes out of the oven and turn with a spatula. Add the courgettes and toss together. Transfer the lamb to the same tray and roast in the oven for 20 minutes for pink, medium lamb.

Take the tray out of the oven. Rest the lamb for 5 minutes and keep the vegetables warm. Carve the lamb into individual cutlets. Divide the vegetables between two warmed plates and top with the lamb. Season with a little salt and pepper and spoon over the mint sauce to serve.

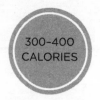

300-400
CALORIES

355
CALORIES
PER SERVING

SERVES 4

PREP: 15 MINUTES, PLUS MARINATING TIME

COOK: 15 MINUTES

INGREDIENTS

75ml dark soy sauce

½ tsp dried chilli flakes

2 tbsp clear honey

20g chunk of fresh root ginger, peeled and cut into very thin strips

2 garlic cloves, thinly sliced

4 spring onions, thinly sliced

4 x 125g fresh salmon fillets (skin on)

1 red pepper, deseeded and thinly sliced

1 orange pepper, deseeded and thinly sliced

175g baby corn, trimmed

150g pack of cooked thick udon noodles

150g mangetout, trimmed

fresh coriander, to garnish (optional)

soy and ginger salmon with noodles

This is a brilliant lunch or supper dish that everyone seems to love and that takes just a few minutes to cook. It's also really delicious served cold as a salad for lunch the following day. You can find cooked noodles in sachets in the Chinese food section of the supermarket.

Mix the soy sauce, chilli flakes, honey, ginger, garlic and two of the spring onions in a medium freezer bag. Add the salmon fillets and toss until well coated in the marinade. Seal the bag and marinate the salmon in the fridge for at least 4 hours or preferably overnight. (It can be left in the marinade for up to 18 hours.)

Preheat the oven to 220°C/Fan 200°C/Gas 7. Scatter the peppers and baby corn over a large non-stick baking tray. Take the salmon fillets out of the marinade and place them, skin side down, among the vegetables. Reserve the marinade and bake the salmon for 10 minutes.

While the salmon is cooking, open the bag of noodles and put them in a colander in the sink. Slowly pour over a kettle full of just-boiled water, lifting the noodles with a fork to separate the strands, and drain.

Take the baking tray out of the oven and add the noodles and mangetout, using tongs or a spoon and fork. Pour over the reserved marinade. Return to the oven for a further 5 minutes, or until the vegetables are tender, the noodles are hot and the salmon is cooked. Sprinkle with the remaining spring onions and coriander to garnish, if you like.

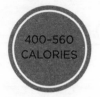

430

CALORIES
PER SERVING

SERVES 2

PREP: 10 MINUTES

COOK: 25 MINUTES

INGREDIENTS

400g baby new potatoes, halved

1 tbsp sunflower oil

¼ tsp dried thyme

¼ tsp dried rosemary

¼ tsp flaked sea salt, plus extra to season

¼ tsp ground black pepper, plus extra to
season

2 x 120g fresh tuna steaks, each about
2cm thick

100g fine green beans, trimmed

250g cherry tomatoes on the vine

1 little gem lettuce, cut lengthways into
wedges

40g pitted black olives in brine, drained

1 tbsp thick balsamic vinegar

warm tuna niçoise

If you like a traditional tuna niçoise, you will love this quick supper dish with fresh tuna, lots of vegetables and a light wholegrain mustard dressing (see page 27). Serve with quartered hard-boiled eggs if you like – each medium egg contains 70 calories extra.

Preheat the oven to 220°C/Fan 200°C/Gas 7. Put the potatoes in a medium roasting tin and toss with the oil. Season with salt and black pepper and roast for 15 minutes.

Mix the dried herbs, salt and pepper. Season the tuna on both sides with the seasoning mix. Take the roasting tin out of the oven and turn the potatoes. Add the tuna and green beans and return to the oven for 5 minutes.

Take the tray out of the oven again and turn all the vegetables and the tuna. Add the tomatoes and bake for a further 3–5 minutes, or until the tuna is cooked to your taste.

While the tuna is cooking, make the dressing (see page 27) if using.

Divide the lettuce between two plates then add the cooked vegetables and olives, top with the tuna and drizzle over the balsamic vinegar to serve.

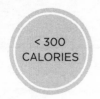
107
CALORIES
PER SERVING

SSERVES 2

PREP: 5 MINUTES

INGREDIENTS

2 tsp white wine vinegar

½ tsp caster sugar

1 tsp wholegrain or Dijon mustard

2 tbsp extra virgin olive oil

flaked sea salt

ground black pepper

Tip: You can also double these ingredients to make a dressing that you can use over a couple of days. It contains a good helping of mustard to complement the flavour of the fish in the warm tuna niçoise recipe (see page 25), so if doubling and using with other salads, keep the mustard to 1 tsp for the best flavour.

vinaigrette

Put the vinegar, sugar and mustard in a medium bowl. Add a pinch of salt and a little freshly ground black pepper. Whisk with a metal balloon whisk to combine, then gradually whisk the extra virgin olive oil into the vinegar mixture until the dressing has thickened slightly. Adjust the seasoning to taste. Pour into a small jug or drizzle directly onto a salad. If serving a little time after it is made, stir well.

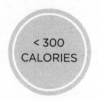
293

CALORIES
PER SERVING

SERVES 2

PREP: 5 MINUTES

COOK: 18 MINUTES

INGREDIENTS

oil, for spraying or brushing

2 reduced fat sausages (10% fat or less)

1 large beef tomato or slicing tomato, halved

10g butter, cut into small pieces

2 large eggs

2 smoked back bacon rashers, trimmed of visible fat

fresh watercress, to serve

flaked sea salt

ground black pepper

one-pan cooked breakfast

It's possible to make really creamy scrambled eggs in the oven if you follow this recipe for the easiest cooked breakfast ever – and there's hardly any washing-up. Look out for 50% reduced-sugar ketchup to serve alongside – it contains 10 calories per tablespoon.

Preheat the oven to 200°C/Fan 180°C/Gas 6. Spray a non-stick baking tray with oil. Place the sausages and a small, shallow ovenproof pie dish on the tray (it will need to hold about 300ml) and bake for 5 minutes.

Take the tray out of the oven, turn the sausages over and add the tomato halves, cut side up, to the tray. Season with salt and pepper.

Put the butter in the warmed pie dish and break the eggs into the dish. Add a pinch of salt and whisk together with a small metal whisk. (If you don't have a small metal whisk, beat the eggs in a separate bowl then add to the dish.) Cover the dish with foil and return the tray to the oven for 5 minutes.

Take the tray out of the oven, turn the sausages and add the bacon. Stir the eggs with a fork then cover with foil again. Return to the oven for a further 5 minutes.

Take the tray out of the oven, turn the sausages and bacon, stir the eggs and return to the oven for a final 3 minutes or until the sausages are cooked and the eggs are scrambled to taste. Remember that the eggs will continue to cook in the heat of the dish.

Divide the scrambled eggs between two warmed plates. Add a sausage, tomato and rasher of bacon to each plate plus a few watercress sprigs. Serve immediately.

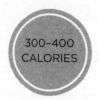

300–400
CALORIES

339
CALORIES
PER SERVING

SERVES 6

PREP: 10–15 MINUTES

COOK: 40–45 MINUTES

INGREDIENTS

375g ready-rolled shortcrust pastry

1 tsp sunflower oil

300g frozen sliced Bramley cooking apples

200g frozen blackberries

1 tbsp cornflour

3 tbsp caster sugar

beaten egg, to glaze

easy apple and blackberry pie

This is a brilliant last-minute pudding, as most of the ingredients can be taken from the freezer and you don't need to be an expert cook to make it. It's heavy on fruit and short on pastry, which cuts the calories and the fat. If you use fresh rather than frozen fruit, you can reduce the cooking time by about 10 minutes.

Preheat the oven to 200°C/Fan 180°C/Gas 6. Unwrap and unroll the pastry onto a large non-stick baking tray brushed lightly with oil.

Mix the frozen fruit, cornflour and sugar together in a bowl or large freezer bag and leave to stand for 5 minutes. Arrange the fruit down the centre of the pastry from one short end to the other, leaving a 5cm gap at each side and at the ends. Pull up the sides of the pastry so it almost covers the fruit and tuck in the ends to seal all the fruit inside.

Brush the pastry all over with the beaten egg and bake the pie in the oven for 40–45 minutes or until golden brown and cooked through. Remove from the oven, and serve hot or cold in slices with fat-free fromage frais or half-fat crème fraiche, low-fat custard or single cream. (Don't forget to add the extra calories.)

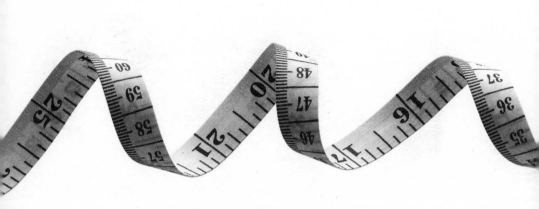

| wok

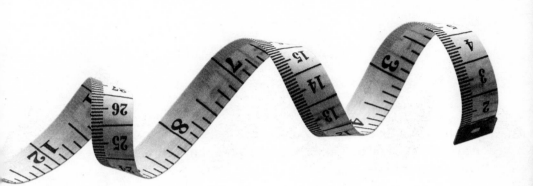

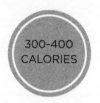

300-400
CALORIES

305
CALORIES
PER SERVING

SERVES 4

PREP: 10 MINUTES

COOK: 10 MINUTES

INGREDIENTS

1 tbsp sunflower oil

3 boneless, skinless chicken breasts (about
450g), cut into roughly 2.5cm chunks

2 medium carrots (each about 100g),
peeled and cut into roughly 5mm
diagonal slices

1 large red pepper, deseeded and cut into
roughly 3cm chunks

150g sugar snap peas, trimmed

3 tbsp Thai sweet chilli sauce

2 tbsp dark soy sauce, plus extra to serve

6 spring onions, trimmed leaving lots of
green, and cut into roughly 2cm lengths,
plus extra to garnish

250g sachet pre-cooked long grain rice

Tip: Look out for sachets of cooked rice in the supermarket – the
rice only needs reheating for a few minutes and is perfect for
one-pan dishes like this.

chilli chicken stir-fry with rice

Thai sweet chilli dipping sauce and soy sauce combine to make a quick and convenient sauce for this colourful stir-fry – and using pre-cooked rice saves using an extra pan.

Place a large non-stick frying pan or wok over a medium-high heat. Pour the sunflower oil into the pan and as soon as it is hot, add the chicken and stir-fry for 2 minutes, or until very lightly coloured all over.

Scatter the carrots, pepper and peas into the pan with the chicken and stir-fry for a further 4–5 minutes, until almost tender.

Pour over the chilli and soy sauces, add the spring onions and toss together for a few seconds, then add the rice and cook for a further 3 minutes, or until the rice and chicken are hot throughout, stirring continuously.

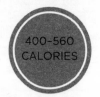

400–560
CALORIES

467
CALORIES
PER SERVING

SERVES: 4

PREP: 10 MINUTES

COOK: 12–15 MINUTES

INGREDIENTS

oil, for spraying or brushing

1 medium onion, finely chopped

600g boneless, skinless chicken breasts (about 4 small breasts), cut into roughly 2cm chunks

2 garlic cloves, crushed or finely grated

100ml white wine

1 chicken stock cube

150ml just-boiled water

3 tbsp cornflour

300ml semi-skimmed milk

2–3 fresh egg lasagne sheets (about 125g), each cut into 3 strips widthways

100g sliced smoked ham, cut into 2cm-wide strips

100g young spinach leaves

100g ready grated mozzarella (from a packet)

20g Parmesan cheese, finely grated

large mixed salad, to serve

Tip: If you can't find fresh lasagne in your local shops, cook dried lasagne in boiling water until almost tender instead.

chicken and ham wok lasagne

It's hard to believe that a lasagne could be cooked in a wok, but it's perfectly possible with this speedy one-pot pasta dish. Use fresh lasagne sheets – you'll find them in the chiller aisle – and freeze any leftover sheets for next time.

Brush or spray a little oil into a large non-stick, flameproof wok and place over a medium heat. Add the onion and chicken pieces and stir-fry for 3 minutes, or until very lightly coloured.

Stir in the garlic then the wine. Crumble the stock cube over and stir until it starts to dissolve. Add the just-boiled water, bring to a gentle simmer and cook for 1 minute.

While the liquid is simmering, stir 3 tablespoons of the milk into the cornflour in a bowl to make a smooth paste. Pour the rest of the milk and the cornflour mixture into the pan with the chicken and bring back to a gentle simmer, stirring frequently. Rinse the pasta strips quickly under cold water.

Add the ham, spinach leaves and pasta to the wok and simmer gently for 5 minutes, stirring frequently until the pasta is tender. Preheat the grill to its hottest setting.

Scatter the grated mozzarella and Parmesan cheese on top of the lasagne. Season with black pepper and grill for 3–5 minutes, or until the cheese is melted and beginning to brown. Make sure your wok doesn't have wooden or plastic handles, so it can go under the grill. Alternatively, transfer the lasagne to a suitable dish before grilling, but make sure you warm the dish before you add the lasagne. Serve with a large mixed salad.

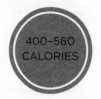

400-560
CALORIES

429

CALORIES
PER SERVING

SERVES 4

PREP: 15 MINUTES

COOK: 40 MINUTES

INGREDIENTS

8 boneless, skinless chicken thighs
(about 675g), trimmed of visible fat
and cut in half

1 tbsp sunflower oil

1 medium onion, roughly chopped

4 garlic cloves, thinly sliced

4 tbsp medium curry paste

2 tbsp cornflour

250ml cold water

400ml can reduced-fat coconut milk

1 tbsp Thai fish sauce (nam pla)

300g potatoes (ideally Maris Piper), peeled
and cut into roughly 3cm chunks

150g fine green beans, trimmed

1 large red pepper, deseeded and cut into
roughly 3cm chunks

1 large green pepper, deseeded and cut into
roughly 3cm chunks

2–3 tbsp fresh lime juice

flaked sea salt

ground black pepper

coconut chicken curry

This creamy curry features both Indian and South East Asian flavours and is inspired by popular chicken curries made in the Philippines. The addition of potatoes, peppers and beans means you don't need to serve it with additional rice or breads.

Season the chicken thighs with salt and pepper. Heat the oil in a large, wide non-stick saucepan or sauté pan and fry the chicken in two batches for 2–3 minutes, until lightly browned. Transfer to a plate and set aside.

Add the onion to the pan and stir-fry for 3 minutes or until it's starting to soften. Stir in the garlic and curry paste and cook for a few seconds more.

Mix the cornflour with 2 tablespoons of the cold water in a bowl to make a thin paste. Pour the coconut milk and remaining water into the pan with the onion and stir in the cornflour mixture and Thai fish sauce.

Return the chicken pieces to the pan along with any resting juices. Add the potatoes, cover loosely with a lid or a large piece of foil and bring to a gentle simmer. Cook over a medium heat for 15 minutes. Remove the lid a couple of times, stir and turn the chicken as it cooks.

When the 15 minutes is up, stir in the beans and peppers. Cover loosely and cook for a further 10 minutes, or until the chicken and vegetables are tender, stirring frequently. Remove from the heat and stir in the lime juice to taste. The curry should taste creamy, but also hot and slightly sour.

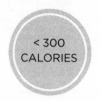

286
CALORIES
PER SERVING

SERVES 4

PREP: 10 MINUTES

COOK: 18 MINUTES

INGREDIENTS

12 ready-made meatballs (about 300g, 20% fat or less)

2 pak choi (each about 100g)

2 medium carrots (each about 100g), peeled and cut into roughly 5mm diagonal slices

1 medium red onion, peeled and cut into 12 thin wedges

1 large red pepper, deseeded and cut into roughly 3cm chunks

150g mangetout, trimmed

5 tbsp hoisin sauce (from a jar)

hoisin meatball stir-fry

This is a stir-fry that's cheap and quick to cook. Meatballs can be fairly high in fat, but that means you don't need any extra fat to stir-fry the vegetables. Serve with a portion of rice or noodles, or just as it is.

Place a large non-stick wok or frying pan over a medium-high heat and add the meatballs. Cook (without additional fat) for 10 minutes, turning regularly until browned all over and cooked through.

While the meatballs are cooking, trim the pak choi and then cut into roughly 2.5cm-wide slices. Separate the green leaves from the whitish stalks. Add the carrots, onion, pepper and the pak choi stalks to the wok with the meatballs and stir-fry for 5 minutes. Add the mangetout and green pak choi leaves and cook for a further 2 minutes.

Spoon over the hoisin sauce and toss with the meatballs and vegetables. Cook for a further minute, stirring and tossing until hot throughout.

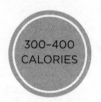

346
CALORIES
PER SERVING

SERVES 4

PREP: 15 MINUTES

COOK: 15–18 MINUTES

INGREDIENTS

500g pork tenderloin (fillet), trimmed and cut into roughly 2cm slices

1 small Savoy cabbage (about 475g)

300ml cold water

1 tbsp sunflower oil

1 medium onion, cut into thin wedges

2 small red eating apples, quartered, cored and sliced

200ml dry cider

2 tbsp cornflour

150ml hot pork or chicken stock (made with ½ cube)

2 tsp wholegrain or Dijon mustard

300g can peeled new potatoes, drained and halved (180g drained weight)

3 tbsp half-fat crème fraiche

flaked sea salt

ground black pepper

Flat-freeze the cooked, cooled pork, vegetables and sauce in two large freezer bags. Thaw overnight in the fridge. Reheat in a large wok over a medium heat, stirring frequently until piping hot.

creamy pork, apples and cabbage

Tender pork in a creamy sauce with sautéed apples, cabbage and potatoes – all cooked in a wok! It's best to get everything ready before you begin to cook, as it doesn't take long.

Season the pork generously with salt and pepper, and put to one side.

Remove any damaged leaves from the cabbage and cut in half. Cut out the tough central core and then thinly shred the leaves. You should end up with about 375g of shredded cabbage.

Place the cabbage in a large non-stick wok on a medium-high heat, pour over 300ml cold water, cover with a lid or a large piece of foil and bring to the boil. Cook the cabbage for 3½–5 minutes, or until just tender, stirring once. Drain in a colander.

Pour 2 teaspoons of the oil into the same wok and place over a high heat. Fry the pork in two batches for 2–3 minutes until well browned on both sides but not quite cooked through. Tip onto a plate, set aside and return the wok to the heat. Add the remaining oil and fry the onion for 3 minutes, then add the apple slices and cook for a further 2 minutes, or until the onion and apples are lightly browned.

Mix 3 tablespoons of the cider with the cornflour in a bowl until smooth. Return the pork to the pan, add the remaining cider, the stock, mustard, cornflour mixture and potatoes. Bring to a simmer and cook for 2 minutes, stirring frequently. Stir in the crème fraiche and season to taste with salt and pepper.

Pile the cabbage on top of the bubbling sauce and cover once more. Simmer for a further 2 minutes, or until the pork is cooked and the cabbage is hot. Serve in wide bowls.

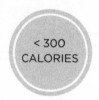

SERVES 2

PREP: 10 MINUTES

COOK: 5 MINUTES

INGREDIENTS

For the wraps

1 little gem lettuce, leaves separated

1 medium carrot, peeled and cut into
  thin sticks

1 red pepper, deseeded and cut into
  thin sticks

2 spring onions, cut into thin sticks

small handful of fresh mint leaves (optional)

small handful of fresh coriander leaves
  (optional)

lime wedges, for squeezing

For the prawns

6 Szechuan peppercorns (Sichuan pepper)
  or 12 black peppercorns

15g chunk of fresh root ginger, peeled and
  cut into fine matchsticks

1 tsp dried chilli flakes, plus a pinch extra
  to serve

200g raw, peeled king prawns, thawed
  if frozen

2 tbsp hoisin sauce

ginger and chilli prawn wraps

If you like Chinese-style duck pancakes, you are sure to enjoy my healthy take on the classic combination. I've used low-calorie prawns and lettuce wraps rather than duck and pancakes, but there's still hoisin sauce for dribbling and crunchy vegetables for piling up on the prawns. It's all cooked in one pan, but you'll need a couple of small dishes for serving the prawns and sauce separately; otherwise, combine them both in the wok and serve on plates with the vegetables.

Separate the lettuce leaves and place them on a serving board or platter. Add piles of the other vegetables to the board and scatter with mint and coriander leaves, if using.

Lightly crush the peppercorns in a pestle and mortar and tip into a non-stick wok or frying pan. Place over a high heat and cook for a few seconds, then add the ginger, chilli flakes and prawns. Stir-fry for 2 minutes, or until the prawns are hot, cooked and pink throughout. Tip into a heatproof bowl and set aside.

Discard any liquid from the pan then return to the heat and add the hoisin sauce and 2 tablespoons of cold water. Heat for a few seconds until thoroughly combined, stirring continuously, then pour into another small heatproof bowl.

Serve the hot prawns in lettuce leaf wraps with the vegetable strips and herbs, drizzled with the warm hoisin dressing. Squeeze over a little lime juice if you like.

Tip: Szechuan peppercorns are mouth-tingling spicy, but black peppercorns work well too.

SERVES 4

PREP: 15 MINUTES

COOK: 15–18 MINUTES

INGREDIENTS

1 tbsp sunflower oil

1 medium onion, thinly sliced

1 red pepper, deseeded and cut into roughly 3cm chunks

1 green pepper, deseeded and cut into roughly 3cm chunks

2 garlic cloves, crushed or finely grated

20g chunk of fresh root ginger, peeled and finely grated

2 tbsp medium curry paste

4 ripe tomatoes, roughly chopped

1 long green chilli, trimmed and thinly sliced

1 tbsp white wine vinegar or cider vinegar

150ml cold water

200ml coconut milk

1 tsp flaked sea salt

1 tsp caster sugar

500g thick, skinless white fish fillet, such as cod, haddock or pollack, cut into roughly 3cm chunks

warmed chapatis (optional)

goan fish curry

I love this curry. It's spicy, sour and sweet, a really great way of incorporating fish into your diet, and it's very quick to cook. If you don't like much heat, deseed the chilli before slicing. Chapatis are low in calories and make a good side.

Heat the oil in a large non-stick wok or frying pan over a medium heat and add the onion. Fry for 3 minutes, stirring until softened and lightly browned then add the pepper, garlic and ginger and cook for a further 2 minutes, stirring.

Stir the curry paste into the pan and fry with the onion, garlic and ginger for a few seconds, stirring continuously. Add the chopped tomatoes and chilli to the same pan and stir in the vinegar and 4 tablespoons of the water. Cook for 3–4 minutes, or until the tomatoes are well softened, stirring frequently.

Pour the coconut milk into the pan and add the remaining water, salt and sugar. Bring to a gentle simmer and cook for 2 minutes, stirring occasionally.

Place the fish on top of the curry sauce, cover and simmer for 3–5 minutes, or until the fish is just cooked. The cooking time of the fish will depend on how large your pieces are and how dense the fish. Give the pan a little shake every now and then as it cooks, but try not to stir, as you could break up the fish. Serve immediately with warm chapatis, if you like, but don't forget to add the extra calories.

Tip: This recipe doesn't use reduced-fat coconut milk, just half a can of the full-fat version. Flat-freeze any leftover coconut milk for up to one month and thaw at room temperature before using the same day.

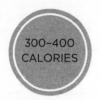

367

CALORIES
PER SERVING

SERVES 4

PREP: 20 MINUTES

COOK: 35–40 MINUTES

INGREDIENTS

1 tbsp sunflower oil

225g paneer, drained and cut into roughly 2cm cubes

1 tsp cumin seeds

2 medium onions, sliced

3 garlic cloves, crushed or finely grated

25g chunk of fresh root ginger, peeled and finely grated

1 long green chilli, finely chopped

1 tbsp medium curry powder

400g can chopped tomatoes

400g potatoes (ideally Maris Piper), peeled and cut into roughly 2.5cm chunks

500ml cold water

½ tsp fine sea salt, plus extra to season

1 tsp caster sugar

100g young spinach leaves

100g frozen peas

ground black pepper

Flat-freeze the cooked and cooled curry in labelled zip-seal bags for up to 1 month. Cook from frozen or thaw in the fridge overnight. Reheat in a large, wide-based saucepan, stirring gently until piping hot.

paneer and vegetable curry

Paneer is an Indian cheese that cooks beautifully and retains its texture. This is one vegetarian dish that even meat lovers will enjoy. It's quite fiery, so if you prefer your curry a little milder, deseed the chilli before chopping.

Place a large non-stick wok or frying pan over a medium heat. Brush with a little of the oil, then fry the paneer in two batches for 3–4 minutes, turning regularly until the cubes are lightly browned. Transfer to a plate, set aside and return the wok to the hob.

Add the remaining sunflower oil to the wok or pan and fry the cumin seeds over a medium-high heat for a few seconds, stirring. Add the onions, garlic, ginger and green chilli and cook for 6–8 minutes, stirring regularly until the onions are well softened. Sprinkle over the curry powder and cook for about 30 seconds, stirring.

Tip the chopped tomatoes into the pan, add the potatoes, water and salt. Season with plenty of black pepper. Bring the sauce to a gentle simmer, stirring continuously. Cover and cook the sauce for about 20 minutes, or until the potatoes are tender. Don't let the sauce boil furiously and stir it frequently as it simmers, especially towards the end of the cooking time.

When the curry sauce is ready, stir in the sugar, the spinach leaves (a handful at a time) and the frozen peas. Cook for a further 2–3 minutes until hot, adding a little extra water if needed, then add the paneer and heat through gently. Check the seasoning – you may want a little extra salt or pepper – and serve.

277

CALORIES
PER SERVING

SERVES 4

PREP: 10 MINUTES

COOK: 12 MINUTES

INGREDIENTS

350g frozen mixed vegetables, such
  as peas, sweetcorn, carrots and beans
125g gram flour (chickpea flour), sifted
20g bunch of fresh coriander, leaves
  finely chopped
1 tsp fine sea salt
1 tsp hot chilli powder
½ tsp ground turmeric
100ml warm water
500–650ml sunflower oil, for frying
cucumber yoghurt (see page 53), mango
  chutney, lime wedges and fresh
  coriander, to serve

Freeze the cooked and cooled pakoras in a freezer bag for up
to 1 month. Reheat from frozen on a baking tray in a preheated
oven at 200°C/Fan 180°C/Gas 6 for about 10 minutes or until
piping hot.

vegetable pakoras

Using frozen vegetables for these pakoras is both cost effective and quick. Serve as a light meal with dips (see minted cucumber yoghurt, see page 53) and a salad, if you like. It might seem strange to include deep-frying in a low calorie cookbook but overall the meal remains low in calories and that's what really counts.

Put the vegetables into a sieve and pour a kettleful of just-boiled water over them. Leave to drain for 2–3 minutes then tip into a large mixing bowl. Add the gram flour, salt, chilli powder and turmeric and toss lightly together. Stir in the warm water, stirring continuously until the vegetables are coated with a thick batter.

Pour the oil into a wok or wide-based saucepan until it is roughly 2.5cm deep. Heat the oil to 160°C on a cooking thermometer. Do not allow the oil to overheat or leave hot oil unattended.

Take a heaped dessertspoon of the batter and drop it very gently and carefully into the hot oil. You will need to push it off the spoon with a second spoon. Continue adding batter until you have 4 pakoras frying at the same time. Cook them for about 3 minutes, turning once or twice with a metal slotted spoon or tongs, until crisp and golden brown.

Lift out of the oil with the tongs or spoon and drain on kitchen paper. Allow the oil to return to the correct temperature and continue cooking the remaining pakoras in two more batches, exactly the same way. Serve warm with cucumber yoghurt, mango chutney (about 50 calories per tablespoon), lime or lemon wedges, and fresh coriander.

< 300
CALORIES

25
CALORIES
PER SERVING

SERVES: 4

PREP: 6-8 MINUTES

INGREDIENTS

$^1/_3$ cucumber

150g fat-free natural yoghurt

10g fresh mint, roughly 4-5 stalks

flaked sea salt

ground black pepper

minted cucumber yoghurt

This is a very versatile dip that goes brilliantly with any spicy foods. I serve it with curries and chillies or as part of a meze-style meal with other dips, cured meats and olives too.

Put the cucumber on a board and grate coarsely. Hold the grated cucumber in your hands over a bowl or the sink and squeeze out as much water as you can. You can also do this in a sieve, pressing down on the cucumber with a ladle. Tip the squeezed cucumber into a bowl.

Strip the mint leaves off the stalks and chop finely. Add to the cucumber and stir in the yoghurt. Season with salt and freshly ground black pepper. Leave for a few minutes to allow the flavours to mingle. If making ahead, cover and chill the yoghurt then stir well before serving. Kept in the fridge, it can be enjoyed for up to 2 days.

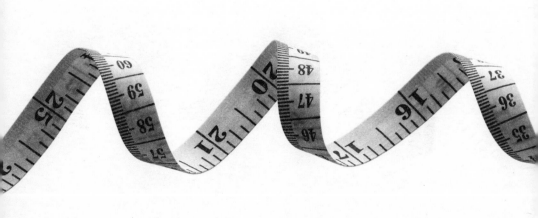

| saucepan

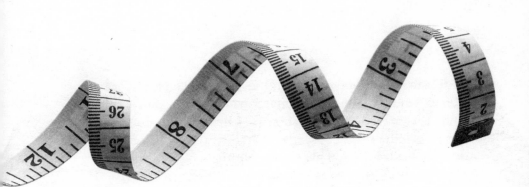

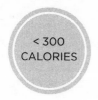

< 300
CALORIES

140
CALORIES
PER SERVING

SERVES 6

PREP: 10 MINUTES

COOK: 35 MINUTES

INGREDIENTS

15g butter

1 tbsp sunflower oil

2 medium onions, roughly chopped

3 medium leeks (about 450g in total), trimmed and thinly sliced

500g potatoes (ideally Maris Piper), peeled and cut into roughly 2cm chunks

1 litre cold water

1 chicken or vegetable stock cube

100ml semi-skimmed milk

flaked sea salt

ground black pepper

Flat-freeze the cooked and cooled soup in labelled zip-seal bags for up to 6 months. Put the frozen soup into a saucepan and thaw gently, stirring as it melts. As soon as all the soup has defrosted, bring to a simmer and cook, stirring frequently, until piping hot. Add a little extra water if necessary. Alternatively, thaw in the fridge overnight and reheat in a saucepan or microwave.

leek and potato soup

Heavy on leeks, cheap and filling, this soup makes for a welcome meal on a cold day and it can be reheated from frozen. When the weather is hot, serve it chilled with a swirl of half-fat crème fraiche and a sprinkling of chives for a delicious vichysoisse.

Melt the butter with the oil in a large non-stick saucepan over a low heat and fry the onions and leeks for 8–10 minutes, stirring frequently until well softened.

Add the potatoes to the pan and stir in the water and stock cube. Bring to the boil, then reduce the heat slightly and simmer uncovered for about 20 minutes, or until all the vegetables are very soft, stirring occasionally.

Remove the pan from the heat and stir in the milk. Remove from the heat and blitz with a stick blender until smooth. (Alternatively, cool for a few minutes then transfer in batches to a liquidiser or food processor and blend until smooth.) Season with salt and pepper to taste and reheat gently, adding extra water if necessary until the right consistency is reached.

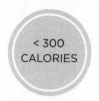

108
CALORIES
PER SERVING

SERVES 6

PREP: 15 MINUTES

COOK: 30 MINUTES

INGREDIENTS

1 tbsp sunflower oil

2 medium onions, roughly chopped

5 medium carrots (about 500g), peeled
and cut into roughly 1.5cm slices

1 sweet potato (about 300g), peeled and
cut into roughly 2cm chunks

2 garlic cloves, thinly sliced

1 tsp ground coriander

$\frac{1}{4}$ tsp hot chilli powder

1.3 litres chicken or vegetable stock (made
with 1 stock cube)

20g bunch of fresh coriander, including the
stalks, roughly chopped

flaked sea salt

ground black pepper

Flat-freeze the cooked and cooled soup in labelled zip-seal bags
for up to 6 months. Put the frozen soup into a saucepan and thaw
gently, stirring as it melts. As soon as all the soup has defrosted,
bring to a simmer and cook, stirring frequently, until piping hot.
Add a little extra water if necessary. Alternatively, thaw in the
fridge overnight and reheat in a saucepan or microwave.

carrot, sweet potato and coriander soup

I'm a huge fan of carrot and coriander soup, and chunks of sweet potato bring a new dimension, making it even more delicious. Blitzing the coriander stalks as well as the leaves adds lots of extra flavour to the soup.

Heat the oil in a large non-stick saucepan and gently fry the onions with the carrots and sweet potato for 10 minutes, stirring occasionally. Add the garlic, ground coriander and chilli powder and cook for a further 30 seconds, stirring continuously.

Pour over the stock and bring to the boil. Reduce the heat to a simmer and cook for about 20 minutes, or until the carrots are very soft, stirring occasionally. Remove from the heat.

Blitz the soup with a stick blender until very smooth. (If you don't have a stick blender, allow the soup to cool for a few minutes then blend in a food processor or liquidiser instead.) Add the coriander and blitz once more. Add a little extra water if needed, until the perfect consistency is reached. Season with salt and pepper to taste. Reheat gently just before serving, stirring continuously.

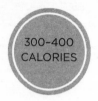

356

CALORIES
PER SERVING

SERVES 5

PREP: 15 MINUTES

COOK: 40 MINUTES

INGREDIENTS

2 tbsp sunflower oil

6 boneless, skinless chicken thighs
 (about 500g), trimmed of visible fat
 and each cut into 3 pieces

2 medium onions, thinly sliced

3 tbsp medium curry paste

2 medium carrots (each about 100g),
 peeled and cut into roughly 5mm
 diagonal slices

½ medium cauliflower (about 300g),
 cut into small florets

100g fine green beans, trimmed and cut
 into 3cm lengths

800ml hot chicken stock (made with
 1 chicken cube)

150g basmati rice, rinsed and drained

150g frozen peas

15g bunch of fresh coriander, leaves
 roughly chopped

fat-free natural yoghurt and mango
 chutney, to serve

Tip: You'll need to add 8 calories for each tablespoon of fat-free yoghurt and 50 calories for each tablespoon of mango chutney.

hob-top chicken biryani

This is a super, really filling dish. I like to serve it straight from the saucepan with fat-free natural yoghurt and mango chutney, plus a generous scattering of chopped coriander.

Heat the oil in a large, wide-based, non-stick saucepan or sauté pan and fry the chicken and onions over a high heat for 8–10 minutes, stirring frequently until the onions are golden brown. Reduce the heat to medium and stir in the curry paste. Cook for 1 minute, stirring continuously.

Add the carrots, cauliflower, beans and stock. Bring to the boil then reduce the heat, cover loosely and simmer gently for 12–15 minutes, stirring occasionally, until the vegetables are just tender.

Remove the lid, add the rice and continue to cook uncovered for a further 10 minutes or until the rice is tender, stirring occasionally and adding the peas after 7 minutes. (Add a splash more water if all the liquid is absorbed before the rice is ready.)

Sprinkle with coriander and serve with fat-free yoghurt and mango chutney (see tip).

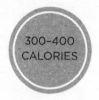

328

CALORIES
PER SERVING

SERVES 4

PREP: 10 MINUTES

COOK: 15 MINUTES

INGREDIENTS

2 medium courgettes, halved lengthways
and cut into roughly 2cm slices

1 red pepper, deseeded and cut into roughly
2.5cm chunks

1 orange pepper, deseeded and cut into
roughly 2.5cm chunks

1 medium red onion, cut into 12 wedges

2 tbsp mild olive oil or sunflower oil

2 boneless, skinless chicken breasts (each
about 175g), cut into roughly 2cm chunks

1 tsp ground coriander

1 tsp ground cumin

1 tbsp harissa paste (from a jar)

4 garlic cloves, thinly sliced

500ml hot chicken stock (made with
1 chicken cube)

150g bulgur wheat, rinsed in a sieve
and drained

2 tbsp fresh lemon juice

flaked sea salt

ground black pepper

fresh coriander leaves, roughly chopped,
to garnish (optional)

lightly dressed green salad, to serve

harissa chicken and bulgur pilaf

Warming harissa paste adds colour and spicy heat to this simple pilaf. It is packed with vegetables, so you'll only need two chicken breasts for a really filling supper.

Put the courgettes, peppers and onion in a large wide-based saucepan or sauté pan and toss with the oil until well coated. Season with salt and lots of black pepper.

Place over a high heat and stir-fry the vegetables for 3 minutes, or until lightly browned but not cooked through. Add the chicken and stir-fry for a further 2 minutes. Stir in the dried coriander, cumin, harissa paste and garlic and cook for 20 seconds, stirring.

Pour over the stock, add the bulgur wheat, and bring to a simmer. Cook for 10 minutes or until the bulgur wheat is tender and the liquid is well reduced and almost all absorbed, stirring frequently, especially towards the end of the cooking time.

Stir in the lemon juice and sprinkle with coriander (if using) just before serving with a lightly dressed green salad.

394

CALORIES
PER SERVING

SERVES 4

PREP: 10 MINUTES

COOK: 35 MINUTES

INGREDIENTS

1 tbsp sunflower oil

12 good quality pork chipolatas

1 large onion, thinly sliced

2 yellow peppers, deseeded and cut into
roughly 3cm chunks

2 medium courgettes, cut into roughly
2cm slices

2 garlic cloves, crushed

¼ tsp dried chilli flakes

1 tsp dried oregano

400g can chopped tomatoes with herbs

400g can cannellini beans, drained and
rinsed

2 tbsp tomato purée

250ml chicken or pork stock (made with
1 stock cube)

150ml red wine or water

flaked sea salt

ground black pepper

fresh flat-leaf parsley, roughly chopped,
to garnish (optional)

simple sausage stew

If the weather turns chilly, this spicy stew is just the thing. Choose chipolata sausages with a high meat content – about 90% is perfect. Using chipolatas means the recipe is easy to divide by four, and the courgettes and beans make it more filling and add extra fibre.

Heat the oil in a large, wide-based non-stick saucepan, sauté pan or flameproof casserole and fry the sausages gently for 10 minutes, turning them every now and then until browned all over. Transfer to a plate and set aside.

Put the onion and peppers in the same pan and fry over a medium heat for 3 minutes until beginning to soften, stirring often. Add the courgettes, garlic, chilli flakes and oregano and cook for a further 2 minutes, stirring.

Stir in the tomatoes, beans, tomato purée, stock and wine or water. Return the chipolatas to the pan. Bring to a simmer. Reduce the heat slightly and leave to simmer gently for 20 minutes, stirring occasionally. Season well with salt and pepper and garnish with chopped parsley (if using) just before serving.

Freeze the cooked and cooled stew in a shallow freezer-proof container for up to 3 months. Thaw overnight in the fridge and reheat in a large saucepan or microwave, stirring frequently until piping hot.

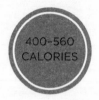

400–560
CALORIES

414
CALORIES
PER SERVING

SERVES 5

PREP: 10 MINUTES

COOK: 40 MINUTES

INGREDIENTS

500g lean minced beef (10% fat or less)

1 large onion, finely chopped

150g closed-cup mushrooms, thickly sliced

2 garlic cloves, crushed

150ml red wine or beef stock

1 litre beef stock (made with 1 beef cube)

400g can chopped tomatoes

2 tbsp tomato purée

1½ tsp dried oregano

250g dried penne pasta

flaked sea salt

ground black pepper

large mixed salad, to serve

Tip: Some supermarket packs of beef are sold as 450g portions, so you can use that instead of 500g. It will reduce the calories by 18 per serving.

Freeze the cooked and cooled pasta and sauce in single-serving freezer-proof containers for up to 1 month. Thaw overnight in the fridge then reheat in the microwave on high for 3–4 minutes per serving, or until piping hot.

bolognese pasta pot

Cook your pasta with the sauce and you'll have a delicious, easy supper and only one pan to wash. Sprinkle with grated Parmesan cheese if you like, but you'll need to add an extra 42 calories for every 10 grams.

Place a large non-stick saucepan over a medium heat and add the minced beef and onion. Cook together for 3 minutes, stirring the beef and squishing it against the sides of the pan to break up the mince. Add the mushrooms and garlic and cook for a further 3 minutes, stirring frequently.

Add the wine or stock, then 500ml of the beef stock. Tip the tomatoes into the pan and stir in the tomato purée and oregano. Season with salt and plenty of black pepper. Bring to a simmer and cook for 15 minutes, stirring occasionally. Remove the lid and stir in the remaining stock. Bring to a simmer and add the pasta, stirring to separate the pieces.

Cook uncovered for 20 minutes, or until the pasta is tender and most of the stock has been absorbed. Stir frequently, especially towards the end of the cooking time. (If your stock is absorbed before the pasta is ready, just add a splash more water and continue cooking.) Adjust the seasoning to taste and serve with a large mixed salad.

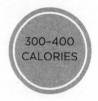

365

CALORIES
PER SERVING

SERVES 4

PREP: 15 MINUTES

COOK: 30 MINUTES

INGREDIENTS

1 tbsp mild olive oil or sunflower oil

1 medium onion, thinly sliced

2 garlic cloves, thinly sliced

1 tsp coriander seeds, lightly crushed

½ tsp dried chilli flakes

1 tsp dried oregano

2 x 400g cans chopped tomatoes
   with herbs

150ml red wine

800ml water

175g dried pasta, such as penne or fusilli

2 medium-large courgettes, halved
   lengthways and cut into roughly 1.5cm
   slices

75g black olives, preferably Kalamata,
   drained and pitted, if preferred

400g thick, skinless white fish fillet, such as
   cod, haddock or pollack, cut into roughly
   4cm chunks

1 tsp flaked sea salt

ground black pepper

chopped parsley leaves, to garnish
   (optional)

italian fish stew

A warming, rich stew with bags of flavour. The pasta cooks in the tomato sauce and the fish is added for the last few minutes. Choose a heavy, wide-based pan so everything cooks evenly, and use short pasta rather than spaghetti or tagliatelle for the best results.

Heat the olive or sunflower oil in a large non-stick, wide-based saucepan or flameproof casserole and gently fry the onion for 5 minutes or until well softened, stirring frequently. Add the garlic, spices and oregano and cook for a few seconds. Stir in the tomatoes, red wine and water and bring to a simmer.

Add the pasta and simmer for 15 minutes, or until it is almost tender, stirring frequently. Add the courgettes and cook for a further 5 minutes, stirring occasionally. Season well with the salt and lots of ground black pepper. Stir in the olives and place the fish pieces on top.

Cover and cook for 5–7 minutes, or until the fish is just cooked and beginning to flake. (The cooking time will depend on the thickness of your fish pieces.) Scatter parsley over the top, if using, and serve. (Watch out for stones if using unpitted olives.)

Tip: You can crush the coriander seeds in a pestle and mortar or use 1 tsp ground coriander instead if you prefer.

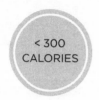

134
CALORIES
PER SERVING

SERVES 6

PREP: 15 MINUTES

COOK: 1 HOUR 10 MINUTES

INGREDIENTS

oil, for spraying

2 medium aubergines (each about 225g), cut into roughly 2cm chunks

1 large red onion, thinly sliced

3 slender celery sticks, trimmed and thinly sliced

3 garlic cloves, thinly sliced

2 x 400g cans chopped tomatoes

50g light soft brown sugar

2 tbsp red wine vinegar

400g can cannellini beans, drained and rinsed

2 tbsp capers (in brine), drained and rinsed

300ml cold water

1 tbsp pine nuts

flaked sea salt

ground black pepper

extra virgin olive oil and basil leaves, to serve

Flat-freeze the cooked and cooled caponata for up to 3 months. Thaw overnight in the fridge and then reheat in a wide-based saucepan or the microwave, stirring frequently until piping hot.

caponata with cannellini beans

Caponata is a thick aubergine stew usually made with lots of olive oil. I've used spray oil for mine, to drastically cut the calories. Cooked long and slow, the aubergines should be silky soft when the caponata is ready. Serve warm or cold with a mixed salad and flatbread, or pile onto hot toasted ciabatta.

Place a large, wide-based non-stick saucepan over a high heat and spray with oil. Add half the aubergine, season with salt and pepper and spray with more oil. Fry for about 4 minutes, or until lightly browned all over, stirring frequently. Tip onto a plate and set aside. Repeat with the remaining aubergine.

Return the saucepan to the heat and add the onion and celery. Spray with more oil and cook for 5 minutes, stirring occasionally. Add the garlic and cook for 30 seconds, stirring, then tip the chopped tomatoes into the pan. Stir in the sugar and vinegar and bring to a gentle simmer. Cover loosely and cook for 15 minutes, stirring occasionally.

Add the aubergines, cannellini beans, capers and water and return to a gentle simmer. Cover loosely again and cook for a further 30 minutes, then remove the lid and cook for 10 minutes more or until very thick, stirring frequently, especially towards the end of the cooking time. Add a splash of water if needed.

Stir in the pine nuts and season with a good pinch of salt and plenty of ground black pepper. Serve warm or leave to cool, cover, chill and eat within 3 days. Drizzle with a little extra virgin olive oil and garnish with basil leaves to serve, but don't forget to add 27 calories for each teaspoon of olive oil.

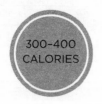

378
CALORIES
PER SERVING

SERVES 4

PREP: 5 MINUTES

COOK: 5 MINUTES

INGREDIENTS

1 small ciabatta loaf (about 350g)

½ garlic clove

1 x full recipe of caponata (see page 71)

small handful of fresh basil, leaves torn
   if large (optional)

1 tsp extra virgin olive oil

ground black pepper

caponata on toast

My caponata (see page 71) is great for serving on toasted ciabatta – a bit like a posh beans on toast, but a lot more filling. You'll need to have the caponata ready, but it freezes beautifully, so well worth making some to have handy if this is the sort of dish you like. It makes a useful meat-free lunch and is a great way to use up aubergines. It also keeps well in the fridge for a couple of days. If you don't have any ciabatta handy, use thin slices sourdough bread instead.

Cut the ciabatta loaf in half horizontally and then cut in half again to make 4 rectangular pieces. Toast on both sides and then rub the cut side with the garlic. If you are using caponata from the fridge, gently warm in a medium saucepan.

Divide the garlic toast between plates and spoon the warm caponata on top. Season with extra coarsely ground black pepper and garnish with basil and drizzle with olive oil if you like.

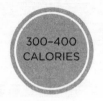

300–400
CALORIES

378
CALORIES
PER SERVING

SERVES 4

PREP: 10 MINUTES

**COOK: 30–35
MINUTES**

INGREDIENTS

1 tbsp sunflower oil

1 medium onion, finely chopped

2 garlic cloves, thinly sliced

1 tbsp medium curry powder

200g dried red split lentils

400ml can reduced-fat coconut milk

½ tsp fine sea salt, plus extra to season

600ml water

500g sweet potatoes, peeled and cut into
   roughly 3cm chunks

1 bay leaf

150g green beans, trimmed and halved

2 tbsp fresh lime or lemon juice

ground black pepper

natural yoghurt, mango chutney, lime
   wedges and fresh coriander leaves,
   to serve

coconut and sweet potato dhal

Lentils are cheap, filling and full of fibre and this simple dhal is quick to cook but tastes very luxurious thanks to the coconut milk. Sweet potatoes and green beans add texture and it's really delicious served hot or just warm with a large crunchy salad, fat-free yoghurt (add 8 calories per tablespoon) and pickles.

Heat the oil in a large non-stick saucepan and fry the onion over a low heat for 5 minutes, stirring frequently until softened and very lightly browned, adding the garlic for the last minute of cooking time. Stir in the curry powder and cook for a few more seconds.

Add the lentils, coconut milk, salt and water. Stir in the sweet potato, add the bay leaf and bring to the boil. Reduce the heat to a simmer and cook the lentils for 15 minutes, stirring frequently.

Add the green beans and cook for a further 10–15 minutes or until the dhal is thick, stirring frequently. Add an extra splash of water if the dhal thickens too much before the lentils are softened.

Stir in the lime or lemon juice and adjust the seasoning to taste. Serve with yoghurt, mango chutney (about 50 calories per tablespoon), lime wedges for squeezing and a sprinkling of coriander.

142
CALORIES
PER SERVING

SERVES 6

**PREP: 5 MINUTES,
PLUS THAWING
AND COOLING TIME**

COOK: 30 MINUTES

INGREDIENTS

250g mixed frozen berries

3 tbsp caster sugar

100g dried tapioca

650ml semi-skimmed milk

250ml water

2 tsp vanilla extract

fruity tapioca puddings

If you like rice pudding desserts, you are bound to love these creamy tapioca puddings. Tapioca is made from the starch of a root vegetable that looks a bit like a yam, and when simmered with milk and vanilla, it makes a comforting dessert with an intriguing texture. You can find tapioca with pudding rice in the desserts section of larger supermarkets.

Put the frozen berries in a freezer bag and add 2 tablespoons of the caster sugar. Thaw at room temperature for 1–2 hours until softened and juicy.

Put the tapioca in a large non-stick saucepan and stir in 500ml of the milk and all the water. Place over a low heat and bring to a gentle simmer. Cook gently for about 25 minutes, stirring frequently, until the tapioca is translucent and the sauce creamy. Stir in the remaining sugar and the vanilla extract. Take off the heat and stir in the remaining 150ml cold milk and leave to cool. (The tapioca can also be eaten warm with cold berries if you prefer.)

Stir the tapioca well and add a little extra water if it's still a little gluey. Divide between six small dishes and top with the juicy berries. Eat the same day or up to a day later if you add the berries just before serving. Cover and keep chilled in the fridge.

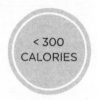

130

CALORIES
PER SERVING

SERVES 8

PREP: 15 MINUTES, PLUS CHILLING AND CHURNING TIME

COOK: 10–12 MINUTES

INGREDIENTS

6 medium egg yolks

50g golden syrup

1 tbsp cornflour

2 tsp vanilla extract or vanilla bean paste

150ml single cream

450ml semi-skimmed milk

freeze-dried strawberry or raspberry pieces
  to serve (optional)

Tip: If the custard begins to look grainy as it heats, it's a sure sign that the eggs are scrambling, so take it off the heat immediately and cool quickly.

lower-fat vanilla ice cream

Finding reduced-fat ice cream that isn't full of artificial additives seems impossible, so I've started making my own. You will need an ice cream maker for this recipe, but borrow from a friend if you don't want to invest in one of your own. My ice cream has roughly 100 calories less per 100 grams than a shop-bought premium ice cream.

Whisk the egg yolks, syrup, cornflour and vanilla in a medium non-stick saucepan using a silicone covered whisk for 1 minute. Pour the cream and milk into the same pan. (If you don't have a silicone whisk, whisk the egg yolks in a bowl and then transfer to the the saucepan.)

Place over a very low heat and cook for roughly 10–12 minutes, stirring continuously with a wooden spoon, until the custard is beginning to thicken enough to coat the back of the spoon. It's important to make sure the mixture does not overheat otherwise the eggs will begin to scramble (see tip).

Remove the pan from the heat and dunk the base of the saucepan into a sink filled with about 6cm of cold water. This will stop the custard continuing to cook. Stir continuously for 5 minutes, then leave to cool in the cold water for a further 30–45 minutes until cold, stirring occasionally.

Put the cooled custard into a pre-chilled ice cream maker. Churn until very thick then transfer to a freezer-proof container, cover and freeze until solid. It could take over 40 minutes to get to an extremely thick consistency, which is what is needed to help ensure the ice cream scoops easily when served.

Remove from the freezer and leave to stand at room temperature for around 10 minutes before serving. Sprinkle with freeze-dried berries if you like.

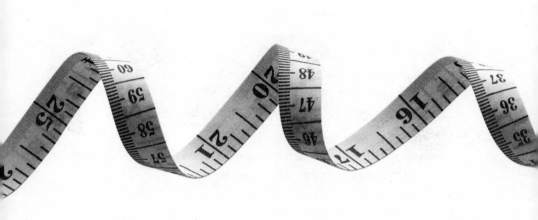

frying pan and griddle

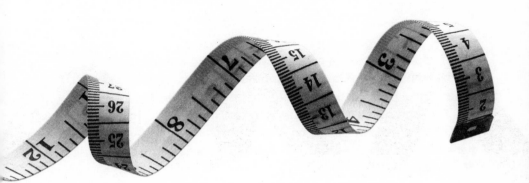

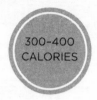

377
CALORIES
PER SERVING

SERVES 4

PREP: 10 MINUTES

COOK: 25–30 MINUTES

INGREDIENTS

25g butter

2 tsp sunflower oil

1 medium onion, finely chopped

400g skinless, boneless chicken breasts
(about 3 small), cut into roughly
2cm chunks

25g plain flour

200ml semi-skimmed milk

150ml hot chicken stock (made with
½ chicken cube)

400g frozen mixed vegetables, such as
broccoli, peas, carrots and cauliflower

3 sheets of filo pastry (each about 45g)

oil, for spraying or brushing

flaked sea salt

ground black pepper

Tip: If you don't have an ovenproof frying pan, transfer the chicken mixture to a shallow ovenproof dish and top with the pastry. Bake for an extra 5 minutes or until the filling is piping hot. Size and shape of filo pastry can vary, but as long as it covers the top of the pie in loosely crumpled heaps the recipe will work perfectly. Your calories may vary slightly depending on the weight of the pastry.

chicken and vegetable frying pan pie

After an exhausting day at work or running around after the family, this is the sort of dish that means you can sit down and relax, knowing there will be very little washing-up at the end of it.

Preheat the oven to 200°C/Fan 180°C/Gas 6. Melt the butter with the sunflower oil in a large, deep ovenproof non-stick frying pan and fry the onion and chicken for 5 minutes over a medium heat until lightly coloured all over, stirring frequently.

Stir in the flour and cook for a few seconds. Slowly add the milk to the pan, stirring continuously, then add the stock and frozen vegetables. Bring to a simmer and cook for 3 minutes, stirring frequently. Season to taste with salt and pepper.

While the chicken and vegetables are cooking, cut each sheet of filo pastry into three pieces, spray or brush lightly with oil and loosely crumple them into small heaps.

Take the pan off the hob and, working quickly, place the crumpled pastry on top of the chicken mixture. Place in the oven and bake for 15–20 minutes, or until the pastry is crisp and golden brown. Take care when you remove the pie as the pan handle will be extremely hot.

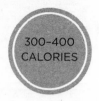

351
CALORIES
PER SERVING

SERVES 2

PREP: 5 MINUTES

COOK: 25 MINUTES

INGREDIENTS

2 boneless, skinless chicken breasts
(each about 150g), cut in half horizontally
to make 4 pieces

1 tbsp sunflower oil

½ medium onion, thinly sliced

2 garlic cloves, crushed or finely grated

227g can chopped tomatoes

2 tbsp tomato purée

300ml chicken stock (made with ½ chicken
cube)

50ml Martini Rosso or Madeira

1 tsp dried oregano

¼ tsp dried chilli flakes (optional)

50g light mascarpone cheese (30% less fat)

small handful of fresh basil, leaves shredded

flaked sea salt

ground black pepper

Freeze the cooked and cooled chicken without the mascarpone
or basil in a freezer-proof container for up to 3 months. Thaw
overnight in the fridge then transfer to a suitable dish and
microwave on high for about 5 minutes. Stir well, top with
mascarpone and microwave for a further 30 seconds or until
piping hot. Garnish with basil.

italian chicken with mascarpone

If you are watching your weight, serve this robust Italian-style dish without additional potatoes, pasta or rice, accompanied by a large mixed salad. It's ready in under 30 minutes and is simple to double up if you are cooking for more than two – or make extra and freeze for another day. If you can't find reduced-fat mascarpone, use the full-fat kind and add an extra 49 calories per serving. Or top with half-fat crème fraiche (24 calories per tablespoon) instead.

Season the chicken breast pieces on all sides with salt and pepper.

Heat the oil in a medium non-stick frying pan (with a base roughly 19cm in diameter). Fry the chicken over a medium-high heat for 3 minutes on each side or until nicely browned and just cooked. Transfer to a plate and set aside.

Add the onion to the pan, reduce the heat and cook for 3 minutes, stirring continuously, until the onion is lightly browned. Stir in the garlic and cook for a few seconds more. (Do not allow the garlic to burn or it will make the sauce taste bitter.)

Tip the tomatoes into the pan, stir in the tomato purée, chicken stock, Martini or Madeira, oregano and chilli flakes, if using. Bring the sauce to a gentle simmer and cook for 10 minutes, stirring frequently.

Place the chicken breasts back into the pan and simmer gently in the hot sauce for 3 minutes. Spoon the mascarpone on top and cook, without stirring, for a further 2 minutes or until the chicken is piping hot and cooked throughout. Remove from the heat and scatter over the basil leaves. Serve with a large mixed salad.

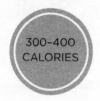

329

CALORIES
PER SERVING

SERVES 2

PREP: 10 MINUTES

COOK: 16–18 MINUTES

INGREDIENTS

2 boneless, skinless chicken breasts
   (each about 150g), cut in half horizontally
   to make 4 pieces

½ tsp dried thyme

¼ tsp dried rosemary

½ tsp flaked sea salt

oil, for spraying or brushing

1 medium red onion, cut into 10 wedges

1 red pepper, deseeded and cut into roughly
   3cm chunks

1 medium courgette, halved lengthways and
   cut into roughly 1.5cm slices

1 tbsp pine nuts

20g Parmesan cheese, thinly shaved with
   a vegetable peeler

large handful of fresh basil, leaves shredded
   if large

2 tbsp thick balsamic vinegar

ground black pepper

pan-fried pesto chicken

I love fresh pesto sauce, but it is usually made with heaps of olive oil, high-fat pine nuts and Parmesan cheese. For this dish, I've included lots of the same flavours but given them a low-calorie twist. If you cut the chicken breasts into four pieces, they cook more quickly and make a serving look very generous.

Sprinkle the chicken breast pieces with the thyme, rosemary, salt and plenty of freshly ground black pepper.

Place a large non-stick frying pan over a medium-high heat. Lightly spray or brush with the oil, add the chicken pieces and fry for 3–5 minutes on each side, until nicely browned and just cooked (there should be no pinkness remaining in the centre when the chicken is cut). Transfer to a plate, cover loosely with foil, and set aside.

Return the pan to the heat, spray or brush with more oil and add the onion wedges, pepper and courgette slices. Stir-fry for 5–7 minutes, or until the vegetables are softened and lightly browned. Add the pine nuts and cook for a minute more, or until lightly toasted.

Return the chicken to the pan and heat through for 1–2 minutes, until hot throughout. Take the pan off the heat and scatter with the Parmesan cheese and basil. Season with black pepper and drizzle with the balsamic vinegar just before serving.

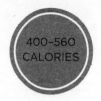

400–560
CALORIES

483
CALORIES
PER SERVING

SERVES 2

PREP: 10 MINUTES

COOK: 7–8 MINUTES

INGREDIENTS

250g lean frying steak (about 1.5cm thick), trimmed of any hard fat and sinew

2 tsp sunflower oil

1 yellow pepper, deseeded and sliced

1 red pepper, deseeded and sliced

8 spring onions, trimmed

4 x 30g mini flour tortillas

4 tbsp soured cream

4 tbsp ready-made tomato salsa

lime wedges, for squeezing (optional)

For the rub

1 tsp jerk seasoning

½ fine sea salt

½ tsp coarsely ground black pepper

Tips: If you can't find jerk seasoning, mix ½ teaspoon hot smoked paprika and ½ teaspoon ground coriander instead. It won't be quite the same, but it will still taste great.

Make your own salsa by mixing chopped tomatoes with finely chopped red onion, finely diced green chilli and freshly chopped coriander leaves.

smoky steak fajitas

Have everything ready before you begin cooking the steak,
and put your extractor fan on full blast. You will need to cook
the meat on a high heat for an authentic over-the-coals
flavour. Frying steaks tend to be cheaper and leaner than
prime cuts and are best cooked rare to medium. Look out for
mini flour tortillas – they are just 30g each and contain around
80 calories rather than 180 calories for a large one.

First, make the rub. Mix together the jerk seasoning, salt and
pepper. Rub the steak all over with half the oil and then the
seasoning mix.

Heat a large non-stick ridged griddle pan over a high heat and
cook the steak for 1½ minutes on each side, until well browned
but not cooked through. Transfer to a board, cover with a piece
of foil and a clean folded tea towel to keep it warm and leave
to rest while you cook the vegetables. (If your steak is thicker
than 1.5cm, you will need to increase the cooking time by
30 seconds or more on each side.)

Return the pan to the heat, add the remaining oil and cook the
peppers and spring onions for about 4 minutes over a medium-
high heat, turning occasionally with tongs until softened and
lightly browned. Transfer to the board.

Meanwhile, heat the tortillas according to the packet
instructions. (Alternatively, heat them on the griddle for a
few seconds on each side.)

Serve the steak and vegetables from the board, piling them
high into warm tortillas with the spring onions and peppers,
soured cream and salsa, with lime wedges on the side if
you like.

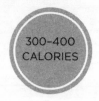

352
CALORIES
PER SERVING

SERVES 5

PREP: 10 MINUTES

COOK: 45 MINUTES

INGREDIENTS

500g lean minced beef (10% fat or less)

1 large onion, finely chopped

½ tsp hot chilli powder

1 tsp smoked paprika

1 tsp ground cumin

1 tsp ground coriander

150ml red wine or beef stock

500ml beef stock (made with 1 beef cube)

400g can chopped tomatoes with herbs

2 tbsp tomato purée

400g can red kidney beans, drained
   and rinsed

flaked sea salt

ground black pepper

For the topping

50g plain tortilla chips

50g sliced jalapeño chillies (from a jar),
   drained and roughly chopped (optional)

50g reduced-fat Cheddar cheese, coarsely
   grated

fat-free fromage frais

chopped fresh coriander (optional)

tortilla chilli pie

For this recipe I've made a lower-fat chilli con carne then topped it with tortilla chips, jalapeño chillies and grated cheese. A quick blast under the grill and it's ready to serve alongside a large mixed salad.

Place a large ovenproof non-stick frying pan over a medium heat and add the beef and onion. Cook for 3–5 minutes, stirring and breaking up the mince.

Add the chilli powder, paprika, cumin and coriander. Fry together for 1 minute, then add the wine followed by the stock. Tip the tomatoes into the pan and stir in the tomato purée. Season with salt and plenty of freshly ground black pepper.

Bring to the boil then reduce the heat, cover loosely and simmer gently for 30 minutes, stirring occasionally. Stir in the red kidney beans, return to a gentle simmer and cook uncovered for a further 10 minutes or until the mince is tender and the sauce is thick, stirring frequently.

Preheat the grill to its hottest setting. Take the pan off the heat and scatter the tortilla chips on top of the chilli, then sprinkle with the jalapeños (if using) and cheese.

Place under the grill for 1–2 minutes, or until the cheese melts. Serve topped with fromage frais and coriander, if you like, and a large mixed leaf salad.

Flat-freeze the cooked and cooled untopped chilli for up to 3 months. Reheat from frozen in a large non-stick flameproof frying pan, adding a little extra water if necessary, until piping hot. Continue as per the recipe.

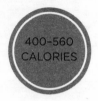

400–560
CALORIES

496
CALORIES
PER SERVING

SERVES 2

PREP: 10 MINUTES

COOK: 28–30 MINUTES

INGREDIENTS

1 medium aubergine (about 250g), cut into roughly 2cm chunks

oil, for spraying or brushing

250g lamb mince (20% fat or less)

½ medium onion, finely chopped

2 garlic cloves, crushed

1 tsp dried oregano

½ tsp dried mint

1 bay leaf

2 tsp plain flour

50ml red wine or extra lamb stock

200ml lamb stock (made with ½ lamb cube)

227g can chopped tomatoes

2 tbsp tomato purée

70g feta cheese, drained, and broken into small chunks

small handful of fresh mint leaves

flaked sea salt

ground black pepper

large mixed leaf salad, to serve

moussaka for two

I like this quick one pan dish of well-seasoned lamb and aubergine better than a traditional baked moussaka. The flavours are rich but fresh-tasting, and the dish looks lovely brought straight to the table.

Put the aubergine chunks in a medium, non-stick frying pan – it should have a base roughly 19cm in diameter and be about 4cm deep – and spray or brush generously with oil. Season with salt and black pepper and place the pan over a high heat. Stir-fry for 3–5 minutes, or until the aubergine is nicely browned but not cooked through. Tip into a medium bowl and set aside.

Put the minced lamb, onion, garlic, oregano, dried mint and bay leaf in the pan used to fry the aubergine and cook over a medium heat for 5 minutes, stirring and breaking up the mince.

Stir in the flour and season with salt and plenty of freshly ground black pepper. Pour over the wine, add the lamb stock, tomatoes and tomato purée. Bring to a simmer and cook for 10 minutes, stirring occasionally. Return the aubergine pieces to the pan and cook for a further 5–10 minutes, or until the lamb is tender, the aubergine is soft and the sauce is thick, stirring occasionally. Drop the feta chunks on top. Cook for a further 1–2 minutes without stirring, until the feta begins to melt. Scatter over the mint leaves and serve.

Flat-freeze the cooked and cooled moussaka without the feta cheese and mint. Reheat from frozen with an extra 100ml water in a large non-stick frying pan for about 20 minutes, stirring frequently, until piping hot. Top with the feta and mint leaves.

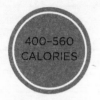

400–560
CALORIES

498
CALORIES
PER SERVING

SERVES 2

PREP: 10 MINUTES

COOK: 25 MINUTES

INGREDIENTS

1 tbsp sunflower oil

2 x 125g salmon fillets

½ medium onion, finely chopped

1 celery stick, trimmed and thinly sliced

2 small carrots, peeled and thinly sliced

50ml white wine

450ml chicken stock (made with ½ chicken
   cube)

250g pouch ready-to-eat puy lentils

10g bunch of fresh flat-leaf parsley, leaves
   roughly chopped, plus extra to garnish

1 tbsp freshly squeezed lemon juice

flaked sea salt

ground black pepper

Tip: The salmon is ready when the flesh begins to flake and looks
opaque. Try not to overcook it or it will become dry.

salmon with puy lentils

Sachets of cooked lentils are handy for one pot meals such as this salmon, cooked with a splash of wine and vegetables. If you aren't keen on fish, use 2 x 125g lean gammon steaks instead and the meal will contain 446 calories per serving.

Pour one teaspoon of oil into a large non-stick frying pan and place over a medium heat. Season the salmon with ground black pepper and fry for 2 minutes skin-side up, until lightly browned. Transfer to a plate and set aside.

Heat the remaining oil in the same pan and gently fry the onion, celery and carrot for 3 minutes, stirring frequently. Stir in the white wine and chicken stock and bring to a gentle simmer. Cook for 10 minutes, or until the carrots are just tender, stirring occasionally.

Stir the lentils and chopped parsley into the pan with the vegetables and season with the lemon juice, a little salt and plenty of ground black pepper.

Place the part-cooked salmon on top of the vegetables and lentils, skin-side down, and simmer for 8–10 minutes, or until the salmon is just cooked. Stir the lentils occasionally and add a little extra water if they become dry. Divide the lentils and vegetables between deep plates, and place the salmon on top (discarding the salmon skin). Garnish with extra parsley just before serving.

371

CALORIES
PER SERVING

SERVES 3

**PREP: 10 MINUTES,
PLUS STANDING**

**COOK: 20–25
MINUTES**

INGREDIENTS

1 tbsp olive oil

1 medium onion, finely chopped

1 small red pepper, deseeded and thinly
   sliced

1 small yellow pepper, deseeded and
   thinly sliced

50g soft cooking chorizo, cut into 5mm
   slices

300g can new potatoes, drained and
   thickly sliced

1 garlic clove, crushed

6 medium eggs, beaten

15g bunch of fresh flat-leaf parsley, leaves
   finely chopped

flaked sea salt

ground black pepper

spanish omelette

It's easy to be a bit sniffy about canned potatoes, but I find them hugely useful for adding to one pot dishes. Here they are combined with lightly sautéed vegetables, chorizo and beaten eggs for an almost authentic Spanish omelette. Serve warm or cold and if you want to make a vegetarian version, simply leave out the chorizo.

Heat the oil in a medium, flameproof non-stick frying pan with a base roughly 19cm in diameter. Add the onion and peppers and cook for 10 minutes over a medium heat until softened and beginning to colour, stirring occasionally.

Add the chorizo and potatoes to the frying pan, season well with salt and plenty of freshly ground black pepper and cook for a further 3 minutes or until hot, stirring frequently. Add the garlic and cook for a few seconds more, stirring.

Mix the beaten eggs and parsley, season with salt and pepper and pour over the vegetables and chorizo. Cook for 5 minutes over a low-medium heat without stirring. Preheat the grill to a medium-hot setting. Place the frying pan under the grill and cook for a further 4–5 minutes or until the eggs are set.

Leave to stand for 5 minutes, then loosen the edges of the omelette with a heatproof palette knife – not metal as it could scratch the non-stick coating – and turn out onto a board. Serve warm in wedges with a large salad. Alternatively, leave to cool then pack into a container, cover and keep in the fridge. Eat within 2 days.

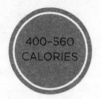

499

CALORIES
PER SERVING

SERVES 2

PREP: 10 MINUTES

COOK: 16 MINUTES

INGREDIENTS

1 tsp sunflower oil

1 red pepper, deseeded and cut into roughly 3cm chunks

1 yellow or orange pepper, deseeded and cut into roughly 3cm chunks

1 medium courgette, cut into roughly 1.5cm diagonal slices

1 medium red onion, cut into 8 wedges with the root intact

½ long red chilli, finely chopped (deseeded first if you like)

1 tbsp extra virgin olive oil

1 tsp fresh lemon juice

227g halloumi cheese, cut into 8 slices

small handful of rocket leaves and fresh mint leaves

ground black pepper

warm griddled halloumi salad

Halloumi is a semi-firm Cypriot cheese that can be sliced and grilled without melting too much. Its salty taste and firm texture means that it is ideally suited to this summery salad.

Place a large, ridged non-stick griddle pan over a high heat for about 5 minutes or until very hot. Put the sunflower oil in a bowl and add the prepared vegetables. Toss gently together.

Griddle the vegetables, in batches if necessary, for about 10 minutes or until softened and lightly browned, turning occasionally. Put in a serving dish or platter and toss with the chilli, olive oil and lemon juice. Season with lots of ground black pepper.

Put the sliced halloumi on the griddle and cook for ½ –1 minute on each side until hot and lightly charred, turning with a spatula or palette knife. Arrange in the dish with the vegetables. Scatter over the rocket and mint leaves and serve while warm.

120

CALORIES
PER SERVING

SERVES 4

PREP: 15 MINUTES

COOK: 15–20 MINUTES

INGREDIENTS

1 ripe medium pineapple (about 1.2kg)

2 tsp sunflower oil

fresh juice of 2 limes (about 4 tbsp)

3 tbsp soft light brown sugar

15g butter

finely pared zest of ½ lime (optional)

caribbean pineapple

Pineapple makes a lovely hot pudding, especially when served with my low-fat 'ice cream' (see page 185). Make sure you cook the pineapple long enough for it to start caramelising in the pan – that way, you don't need to add too much sugar. The calorie count here is for the pineapple only.

Put the pineapple on a board and cut off the top and bottom. Next, cut off all the thick skin and cut out any prickly 'eyes'. Cut the pineapple in half lengthways and then cut each half into 6–8 long slices and cut out the tough central core.

Heat 1 teaspoon of the oil in a large non-stick frying pan and fry half the pineapple slices for 3–4 minutes on each side over a medium-high heat until hot and lightly browned.

Transfer to a plate then add the remaining oil and pineapple to the pan and cook in exactly the same way. Transfer to the same plate as the first batch and return the pan to the heat.

Add the lime juice, butter and sugar to the pan and cook for 1–2 minutes, stirring continuously, until the sugar dissolves and the sauce becomes syrupy. Return the pineapple to the pan and heat through for 1–2 minutes, turning it in the hot sauce.

Divide the hot pineapple and sauce between plates and sprinkle with finely pared or grated lime zest, if you like. Serve with scoops of low-fat 'ice cream' (see page 185). Alternatively, a dribble of chilled single cream goes well, but you'll need to add an extra 29 calories for each tablespoon.

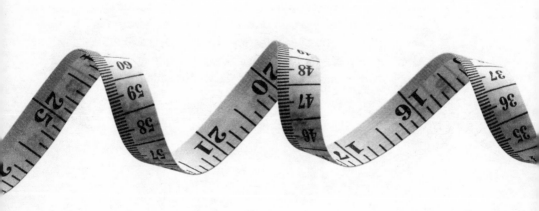

ovenproof dish

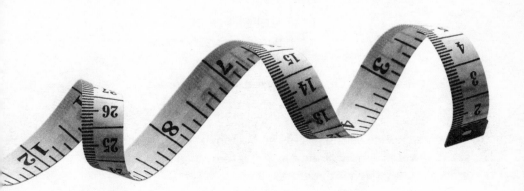

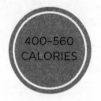

400–560
CALORIES

420
CALORIES
PER SERVING

SERVES 4

PREP: 15 MINUTES

COOK: 1 HOUR

INGREDIENTS

10g dried porcini mushrooms

250ml just-boiled water

1 medium onion, finely chopped

250g closed-cup mushrooms, sliced

2 garlic cloves, very thinly sliced

oil, for spraying or brushing

3 small boneless, skinless chicken breasts
(about 450g total weight), cut into
roughly 2cm chunks

200g Arborio (risotto) rice

100ml Madeira or extra stock

350ml hot chicken stock (made with
1 chicken cube)

50g Parmesan or Grana Padano cheese,
finely grated

flaked sea salt

ground black pepper

fresh flat-leaf parsley, roughly chopped, to
garnish (optional)

large mixed salad, to serve

Tip: If you notice a little grit at the bottom of your mushroom soaking water, simply strain the liquid through a fine muslin or brand new kitchen cloth before using.

baked chicken and mushroom risotto

This full-flavoured risotto is quick to assemble and can be left to cook in the oven, so you don't need to stand stirring it for ages. The dried mushrooms give it a rich, luxurious taste; you will find them in larger supermarkets. Serve this dish with a large mixed salad.

Preheat the oven to 200°C/Fan 180°C/Gas 6. Put the dried mushrooms in a measuring jug and add the water. Leave to stand for about 20 minutes.

Meanwhile, put the onion, fresh mushrooms and garlic in a 3 litre shallow ovenproof dish – a lasagne dish is ideal. Spray or brush with oil and season with salt and plenty of black pepper. Cook in the oven for 15 minutes until softened.

Strain and roughly chop the dried mushrooms, reserving the soaking water. Take the baking dish out of the oven and add the chicken, rice, Madeira or stock, soaked chopped mushrooms and their liquor. Pour over the chicken stock, stir well and cover the dish tightly with foil. Return to the oven for 30 minutes.

Take the dish out of the oven, remove the foil and stir. Cover and return to the oven for a further 10 minutes, or until most of the liquid has been absorbed and the rice is tender. Remove the foil once more, stir in the grated cheese and adjust the seasoning to taste. Scatter with chopped parsley if you like. Serve with a large mixed salad.

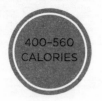

416
CALORIES
PER SERVING

SERVES 2

PREP: 10 MINUTES

COOK: 35 MINUTES

INGREDIENTS

2 parsnips (each about 150g), peeled and
  cut into short batons, about 1.5cm wide
  and 3–4cm long

2 carrots (each about 100g), peeled and cut
  into short batons, about 1.5cm wide and
  2–3cm long

1 tbsp olive oil

1 tbsp clear honey

¼–½ tsp dried chilli flakes (adjust quantity
  depending on taste)

125ml hot vegetable or chicken stock
  (made with ½ vegetable or chicken cube)

75g dried, uncooked couscous

1 tbsp fresh lemon juice

20g bunch of fresh flat-leaf parsley, leaves
  roughly chopped

100g cooked beetroot, drained and cut into
  wedges

50g soft, rindless goat's cheese, cut into
  small pieces

flaked sea salt

ground black pepper

couscous with roasted roots, honey and goat's cheese

A colourful and filling salad with lots of lovely flavours. I like it served warm, but it's also great for packed lunches and will serve four people as an accompaniment.

Preheat the oven to 200°C/Fan 180°C/Gas 6. Scatter the parsnips and carrots over the base of a small, shallow ovenproof dish – it will need to hold about 1 litre – and drizzle with the olive oil. Season with a little salt and lots of ground black pepper and roast for 20 minutes.

Take the dish out of the oven, drizzle the vegetables with the honey and sprinkle with the chilli flakes. Turn to lightly coat, then return to the oven for a further 10 minutes, or until golden and sticky. Tip into a heatproof bowl and set aside.

Pour the vegetable or chicken stock into the ovenproof dish and stir in the couscous. Cover with foil and return the dish to the oven for 5 minutes. Remove the foil, sprinkle over the lemon juice and most of the parsley and fluff up with a fork. Season with salt and pepper. Return the cooked vegetables to the dish and toss together with the couscous.

Scatter the beetroot and goat's cheese on top. Garnish with the reserved parsley and serve warm.

Tip: It's best to use vacuum packed beetroot without vinegar for this recipe (you'll find it with the salad ingredients in the supermarket) but beetroot from a jar can be used too.

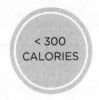

273
CALORIES
PER SERVING

SERVES 4

PREP: 15 MINUTES

COOK: 50 MINUTES

INGREDIENTS

4 medium courgettes (each about 200g),
cut in half lengthways and seeds scooped
out with teaspoon

oil, for spraying or brushing 250g minced
lamb (20% fat or less)

75g bulgur wheat (uncooked)

1 small red pepper, deseeded and cut into
roughly 1.5cm chunks

6 sun-dried tomato pieces, drained and
finely chopped

1 medium onion, very finely chopped

2 garlic cloves, crushed or finely grated

2 tbsp harissa paste (preferably rose
harissa)

1 tsp ground cumin

1 tsp ground coriander

finely grated zest and juice of 1 lemon

20g bunch of fresh mint, leaves finely
chopped, plus extra to garnish

150ml hot lamb stock (made with
½ lamb cube)

4 tbsp fat-free natural yoghurt

1 tbsp pomegranate molasses or thick
balsamic vinegar

ground black pepper

flaked sea salt

spiced lamb-stuffed courgettes

These courgettes are stuffed with minced lamb, spices and bulgur wheat. When baked with a little stock, the wheat softens and expands, making a really delicious supper dish that's great served straight from the oven with spoonfuls of natural yoghurt and a drizzle of pomegranate molasses or thick balsamic vinegar. If you can buy 10% fat lean minced lamb you will save about 51 calories per portion.

Preheat the oven to 220°C/Fan 200°C/Gas 7. Place the halved courgettes fairly tightly together, cut-side up, in a single layer in a shallow ovenproof dish or baking tray. Spray or brush with a little oil, season with salt and pepper and bake for 20 minutes.

To make the stuffing, mix the lamb, bulgur wheat, red pepper, tomato, onion, garlic, harissa, spices, lemon zest and juice, chopped mint leaves and stock. Season with lots of freshly ground black pepper and a little salt.

Take the courgettes out of the oven and spoon the stuffing loosely into the cavities. Cover the dish with foil and bake for 20 minutes. Remove the foil and cook for a further 10 minutes or until the courgettes are softened and the topping is golden and tender. Spoon over the yoghurt, scatter with extra mint leaves and drizzle over the pomegranate molasses or thick balsamic vinegar. Serve hot with a large mixed salad.

254

CALORIES
PER SERVING

SERVES 4

PREP: 10 MINUTES, PLUS COOLING TIME

COOK: 45 MINUTES

INGREDIENTS

oil, for spraying or brushing

2 fresh salmon fillets (each about 125g)

250g asparagus spears (not too thick), trimmed and halved

2 spring onions, trimmed and thinly sliced

20g cornflour

1 tbsp semi-skimmed milk

3 large eggs

200g half-fat crème fraiche

10g bunch of fresh dill, leaves roughly chopped

flaked sea salt

ground black pepper

Tip: Use a ceramic quiche dish for this recipe if you like – it should be about 22cm in diameter and about 4cm high.

salmon and asparagus crustless quiche

Making a quiche without a pastry crust may seem a little odd, but it works well and drastically reduces the calories. Serve in wedges with a mixed salad if you like.

Preheat the oven to 200°C/Fan 180°C/Gas 6. Spray or brush a shallow round ceramic pie dish with oil and place the salmon fillets in it, skin-side down and at least 5cm apart.

Scatter the asparagus and spring onions around the salmon and season with black pepper. Spray or brush with a little more oil and cover the dish with foil. Bake for 12–15 minutes, or until the salmon is just cooked and flakes easily when prodded with a fork.

Take the dish out of the oven and turn the fish over. Remove the skin and flake the fish into large pieces with a couple of forks. Make sure that the fish, spring onions and asparagus are evenly distributed. Reduce the oven temperature to 180°C/Fan 160°C/Gas 4.

Mix the cornflour and milk in a bowl until smooth, then add the eggs, one at a time, and beat together well. (If lumps remain, use a whisk rather than a wooden spoon.) Stir in the crème fraiche and dill. Season well with salt and pepper.

Pour the egg mixture over the salmon and bake for about 30 minutes, or until just set. Leave to cool for at least 15 minutes before cutting into wedges to serve.

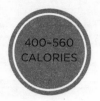

416

CALORIES
PER SERVING

SERVES 2

PREP: 10 MINUTES

COOK: 30 MINUTES

INGREDIENTS

1 orange or yellow pepper, deseeded and
cut into roughly 3cm chunks

1 medium red onion, peeled and cut into
thin wedges

1 medium courgette, trimmed and cut into
roughly 1.5cm slices

oil, for spraying or brushing

1 small lemon

50g soft cooking chorizo, cut into 5mm
slices

2 x 150g skinless thick white fish fillets,
such as cod, haddock or pollack

200g cherry tomatoes, on the vine if
possible

good pinch smoked paprika

1 tbsp extra virgin olive oil

400g can butter beans, drained and rinsed

flaked sea salt

ground black pepper

spanish baked fish with chorizo

A lovely, lightly-spiced cod dish that's perfect if you aren't a confident cook but want to try your hand at cooking fish. It's low in calories but has heaps of flavour and is very filling thanks to all the vegetables and beans. The combination of fish and spicy Spanish sausage works particularly well.

Preheat the oven to 220°C/Fan 200°C/Gas 7. Put the pepper, onion and courgette in a shallow ovenproof dish, spray or brush with a little oil, season with salt and black pepper and bake for 15 minutes.

Cut the lemon in half and cut each half into four chunks. Take the vegetables out of the oven and stir in the chorizo and half the lemon pieces. Place the fish and tomatoes on top of the vegetables.

Squeeze the remaining lemon chunks over the top. Season the fish with salt and pepper and sprinkle with paprika.

Return to the oven and bake for 12 minutes. Take the dish out of the oven and carefully stir the beans into the vegetables and chorizo without disturbing the fish too much.

Return to the oven for a further 5 minutes, or until the beans are hot and the fish is just cooked (this will depend on thickness of the fillets). Serve with a lightly dressed green salad.

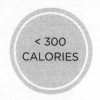

104
CALORIES
PER SERVING

SERVES 6

PREP: 10 MINUTES

COOK: 1 HOUR

INGREDIENTS

3 large red peppers

1 large egg

1 yellow or orange pepper, deseeded
and diced

150g button mushrooms, thinly sliced

50g frozen peas

6 spring onions, trimmed and thinly sliced

2 garlic cloves, crushed or finely grated

150g cold, cooked long grain rice (from
a sachet or home-cooked)

2 tbsp dark soy sauce, plus extra to serve

½ tsp dried chilli flakes

flaked sea salt

freshly ground black pepper

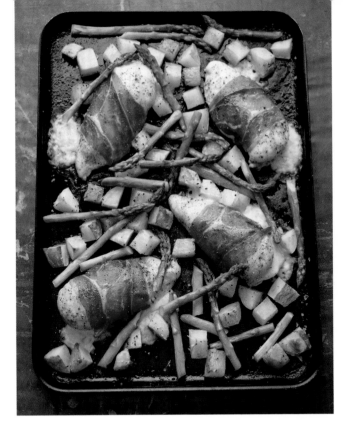

2 = 300–400
CALORIES

quick cheesy
chicken
and ham
(page 3)

2 = 300–400
CALORIES

chilli chicken
stir-fry
with rice
(page 35)

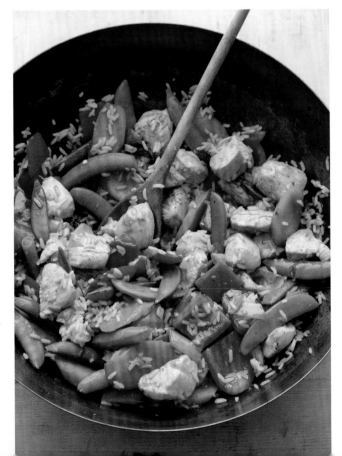

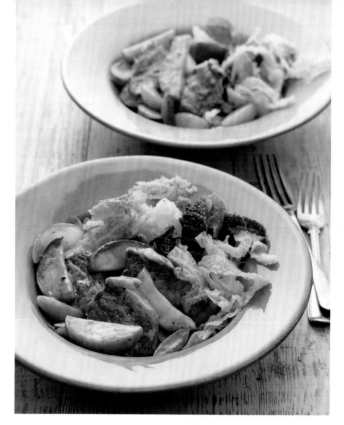

2 = 300–400
CALORIES

creamy pork,
apples and
cabbage
(page 43)

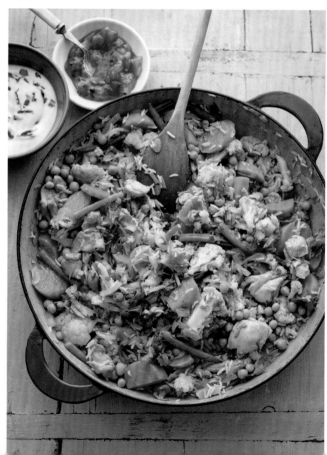

2 = 300–400
CALORIES

hob-top
chicken
biryani
(page 61)

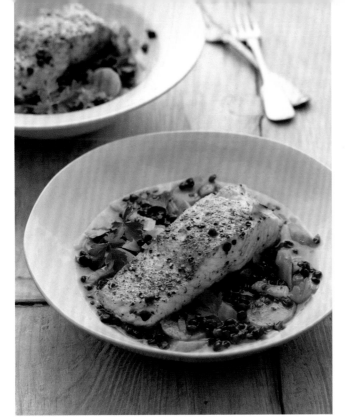

3 = 400–560 CALORIES

salmon with
Puy lentils
(page 95)

3 = 400–560
CALORIES

warm
griddled
halloumi
salad
(page 99)

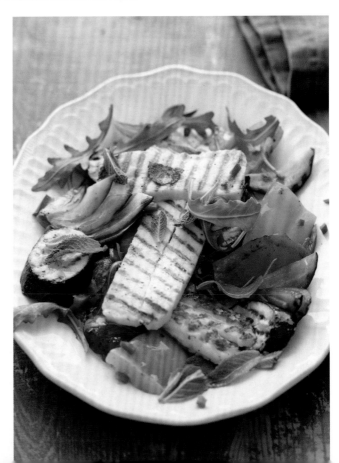

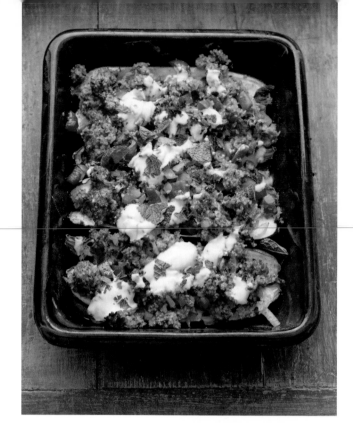

1 = <300 CALORIES

spiced
lamb-stuffed
courgettes
(page 109)

3 = 400-560
CALORIES

spanish
baked fish
with chorizo
(page 113)

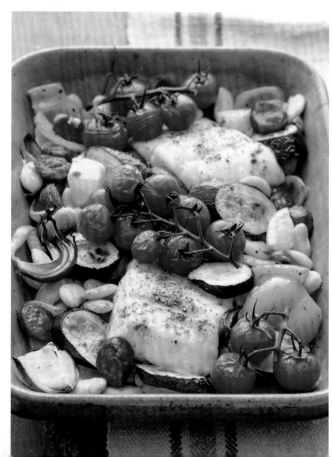

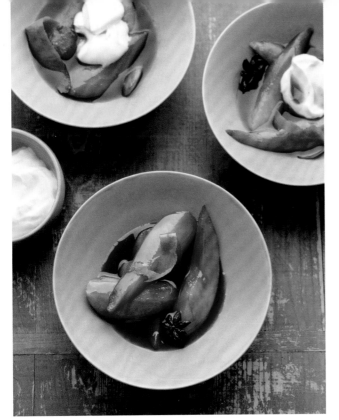

1 = <300 CALORIES

mulled pears

(page 147)

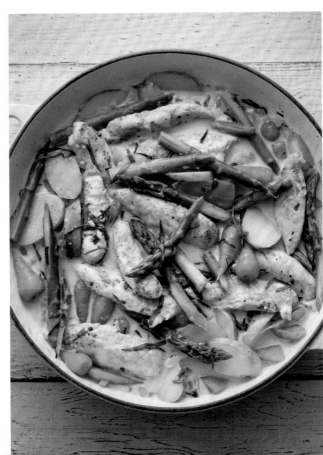

2 = 300–400 CALORIES

tarragon chicken

(page 125)

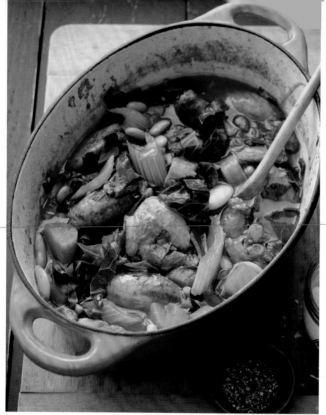

3 = 400–560
CALORIES

simple
cassoulet
(page 127)

3 = 400–560
CALORIES

pibil pulled
pork tacos
(page 139)

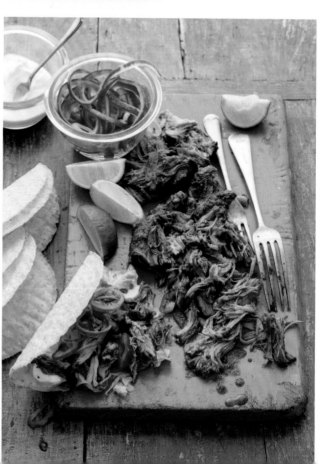

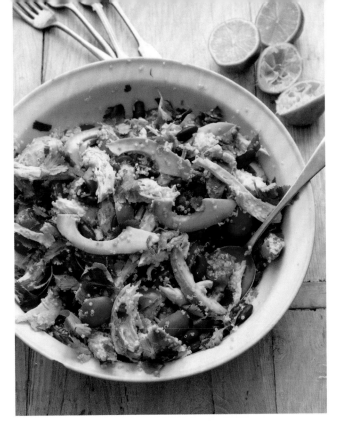

2 = 300–400 CALORIES

Chicken, quinoa, avocado and chilli salad

(page 151)

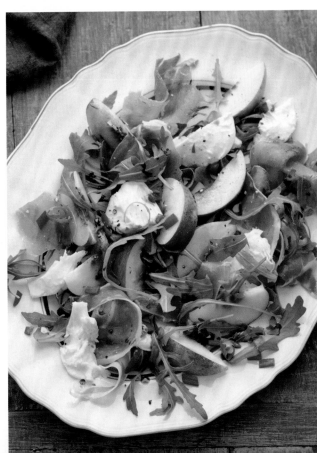

2 = 300–400 CALORIES

nectarine, prosciutto and mozzarella salad

(page 157)

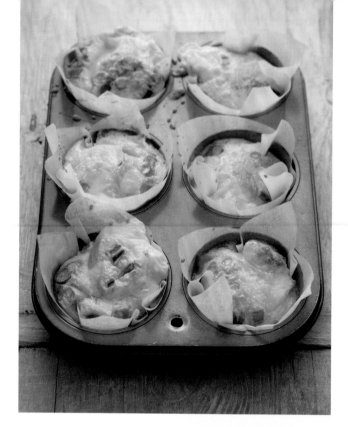

1 = <300
CALORIES

smoked
salmon
breakfast
muffins
(page 169)

1 = <300
CALORIES

milk chocolate
pots
(page 177)

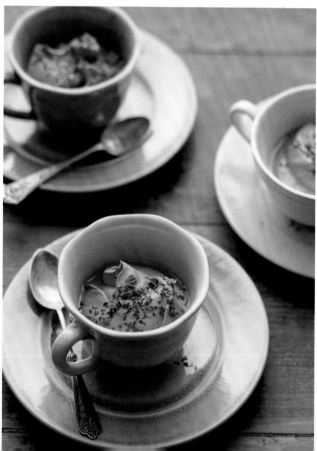

chinese rice-stuffed peppers

A simple, vegetable-packed dish with Chinese flavours. Serve half a pepper with a large mixed salad for a light supper, or two halves for a more filling meal.

Preheat the oven to 200°C/Fan 180°C/Gas 6. Cut the red peppers in half from stem to base and scoop out all the seeds. Place in a single layer, cut side up, in a shallow ovenproof dish – a lasagne dish is ideal. Cut a thin sliver off the base of any peppers that don't sit flat so they hold the filling without tipping. Bake for 20 minutes.

Beat the egg in a medium bowl and stir in the diced yellow or orange pepper, mushrooms, peas, spring onions and garlic. Add the rice, soy sauce and chilli flakes and season with salt and pepper and stir until combined.

Pile the rice mixture into the peppers, cover the dish tightly with foil and bake for 40 minutes, or until piping hot. Serve with more soy sauce for drizzling.

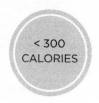

< 300 CALORIES

208
CALORIES
PER SERVING

SERVES 4

PREP: 5 MINUTES

COOK: 30 MINUTES

INGREDIENTS

100g mixed dried fruit

20g flaked almonds

finely grated zest of 1 lemon

3 medium Bramley cooking apples
  (each about 275g)

3 tbsp fresh lemon juice

1 tbsp maple syrup or clear honey

25g butter

fat-free fromage frais or half-fat crème
  fraiche, to serve

Tip: If you want to cut the calories further, leave out the butter and save 46 calories per serving. If the apples begin to scorch before they are completely soft, simply cover the dish with foil and continue baking.

easy baked apples

Baked apples make a great low-calorie pudding, but unless you have an apple corer and spare time for stuffing, they can be a bit of a hassle. My recipe simply cuts the apples into quarters and bakes them on top of mixed dried fruit and flaked almonds. It's much quicker and, I think, more delicious.

Preheat the oven to 200°C/Fan 180°C/Gas 6. Mix the dried fruit, flaked almonds and lemon zest in a small ovenproof dish with a base roughly 21cm in diameter.

Cut the apples into quarters and remove the cores. Place the apples on top of the dried fruit. The apple pieces should sit in a single layer, skin-side up and cover the dried fruit so it doesn't burn.

Drizzle with the lemon juice and maple syrup or honey, dot with butter and bake uncovered for 30 minutes, or until the apples are very tender. Serve with fat-free fromage frais or half-fat crème fraiche, but don't forget to add the extra calories.

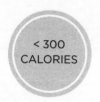

< 300
CALORIES

251

CALORIES
PER SERVING

SERVES 6

PREP: 10 MINUTES

COOK: 35 MINUTES

INGREDIENTS

4 firm ripe nectarines (about 450g total
weight)

150g fresh blueberries

For the topping

50g caster sugar

50ml semi-skimmed milk

1 tsp vanilla extract

50g unsalted butter, well softened

2 medium eggs

150g self-raising flour

1 tsp baking powder

Tip: Peaches make a great alternative to nectarines and contain a
similar number of calories. Prepare them in exactly the same way
as the nectarines.

nectarine and blueberry muffin cobbler

When we first made this in the test kitchen, we thought it tasted just like a warm blueberry muffin – hence the name! The light, fluffy topping is perfect with the juicy nectarines and blueberries.

Take a nectarine and, holding it carefully, cut out slices from top to bottom towards the stone with a small knife, working your way around the whole fruit. Drop the slices into a shallow ovenproof dish, which holds roughly 1.75 litres. You should end up with roughly 8 slices. Discard the stone.

Slice the remaining fruit. Toss the slices with half the blueberries. Preheat the oven to 190°C/Fan 170°C/Gas 5.

To make the topping, put the caster sugar in a large, thick zip-seal freezer bag and add the milk, vanilla extract, butter, eggs, flour and baking powder. Seal the bag and mix the ingredients, squishing and pressing together from outside the bag until thoroughly combined. This will take 2–3 minutes. (You can also mix the ingredients in a food processor or a bowl with a spoon or an electric whisk until smooth.)

Add the rest of the blueberries and mix until lightly combined. Squeeze the open bag over the nectarines, and cover them roughly with the cake batter. Spread it to the sides but don't worry if there are a few gaps.

Bake for 35 minutes, or until the fruit is tender and the topping is risen and golden brown. Serve warm with low-fat custard, half-fat crème fraiche or single cream, but don't forget to add the extra calories.

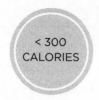

173
CALORIES
PER SERVING

SERVES 12

PREP: 10 MINUTES

COOK: 1–1¼ HOURS

INGREDIENTS

oil, for spraying or brushing

3 very ripe bananas (about 300g peeled weight)

3 medium eggs

1 tsp ground mixed spice

5 tbsp sunflower oil

15g soft light brown sugar

250g self-raising flour

1 tsp baking powder

50g sultanas

Tip: Make sure you use a strong, thick freezer bag to mix the ingredients or the plastic could split. You can also combine the cake ingredients in a bowl with an electric whisk until thick and then add the sultanas.

Freeze the cooked and cooled cake wrapped in foil, and placed in a large freezer bag for up to 1 month. Unwrap and thaw at room temperature for about 3 hours before serving.

quick-mix banana and sultana cake

You can mix the batter for this simple cake in a freezer bag to save time and washing-up! Choose naturally sweet overripe bananas for the best results.

Preheat the oven to 180°C/Fan 160°C/Gas 4. Line the base and sides of a 20cm springclip cake tin with baking parchment and lightly grease with a little oil.

Peel the bananas and cut them into short lengths. Put them in a large, thick freezer bag and squish and press the outside of the bag with your hands until the bananas are mushy.

Add the eggs, mixed spice, sunflower oil, sugar, flour and baking powder and continue to squash, squish and press until you have a thick, almost smooth batter. This will take about 4–5 minutes. Add the sultanas and mix until just combined.

Open the bag and squeeze the cake batter into the prepared tin. Bake for 1–1¼ hours, or until a skewer inserted into the centre of the cake comes out clean. Leave the cake to cool in the tin, then remove and peel off the parchment. Cut into thin wedges to serve.

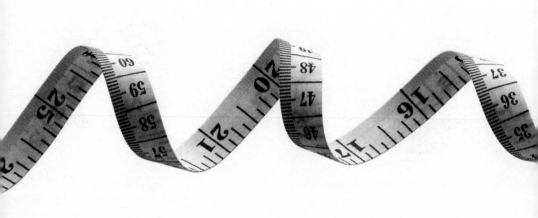

casserole

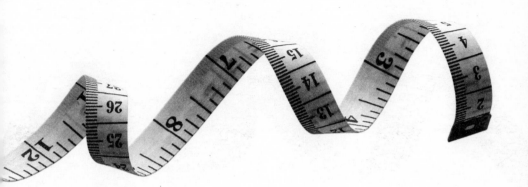

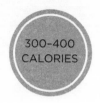

300-400
CALORIES

321
CALORIES
PER SERVING

SERVES 4

PREP: 15 MINUTES

**COOK: 30–35
MINUTES**

INGREDIENTS

400g boneless, skinless chicken breast
 mini fillets

20g butter

1 tsp sunflower oil

1 small onion, finely chopped

1 garlic clove, finely chopped

100ml white wine

500ml chicken stock (made with ½ chicken
 cube)

300g new potatoes, such as Charlotte,
 cut into 1cm slices

300g small carrots, such as Chantenay,
 scrubbed or peeled and halved
 lengthways if thick

small bunch (roughly 15g) of fresh tarragon

250g slender asparagus spears, trimmed
 and halved

3 tbsp double cream

flaked sea salt

ground black pepper

tarragon chicken

Chicken breasts and colourful vegetables are cooked in a light tarragon-infused sauce. I use chicken mini fillets as they're quite cheap, are easy to cook and require no preparation, but you could use sliced boneless chicken breasts instead.

Season the chicken fillets all over with a little flaked sea salt and plenty of freshly ground black pepper. Melt the butter with the oil in a large, shallow flameproof casserole or non-stick sauté pan and fry the chicken fillets for 2–3 minutes on each side over a medium-high heat until golden brown and cooked through. Transfer to a plate and set aside.

Add the onion and garlic to the pan and cook for 2–3 minutes, stirring frequently until the onion is softened and beginning to colour. (Take care not to let the garlic burn or it will taste bitter.) Pour the wine into the pan and let it bubble furiously for a few seconds, then stir in the stock, potatoes, carrots and 2 tarragon sprigs. Cover the pan loosely and simmer very gently for 15 minutes, or until the potatoes are just cooked.

Increase the heat and add the asparagus to the pan. Bring the cooking liquor to the boil and cook the asparagus for about 5 minutes or until almost tender. While the asparagus is cooking, strip the leaves from the remaining tarragon sprigs and chop them roughly.

Stir the cream and chopped tarragon into the sauce and simmer for a further 2 minutes, stirring occasionally. Return the chicken to the pan and heat through for 1–2 minutes or until completely hot throughout. Season to taste and serve immediately.

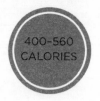

400–560
CALORIES

480
CALORIES
PER SERVING

SERVES 5

PREP: 15 MINUTES

COOK: 1 HOUR

INGREDIENTS

oil, for spraying or brushing

6 herby sausages (at least 85% meat)

1 medium onion, thinly sliced

2 garlic cloves, crushed or finely grated

2 lean smoked back bacon rashers, cut into roughly 1.5cm slices

6 boneless, skinless chicken thighs (about 500g), trimmed of visible fat and cut into three

3 celery sticks, trimmed and cut into roughly 2cm diagonal slices

3 medium carrots, peeled and cut into roughly 2cm diagonal slices

400g can chopped tomatoes

150ml red wine or water

300ml chicken stock (made with 1 chicken cube)

½ tsp dried chilli flakes

1 bay leaf

400g can cannellini or kidney beans, drained and rinsed

400g can butter beans, drained and rinsed

150g baby spring greens or kale, trimmed and thickly shredded

flaked sea salt

ground black pepper

simple cassoulet

This is one of those dishes that everyone seems to like. It's a simple combination of tender chicken thighs and sausages in a rich tomato sauce with canned beans and vegetables – perfect for a weekend lunch, but easy enough for a mid-week supper too.

Spray or brush a large flameproof casserole with oil. Add the sausages to the pan and cook over a medium heat for 10 minutes, turning occasionally until browned on all sides. Take the sausages out of the casserole and put them on a board.

Preheat the oven to 200°C/Fan 180°C/Gas 6. Add the onion to the casserole and cook for 5 minutes, stirring frequently until softened and lightly browned. Add the garlic, bacon and chicken pieces to the pan with the onions and cook for 3–5 minutes, turning the chicken twice until very lightly coloured all over.

Cut the sausages into three pieces and return them to the pan, with the celery, carrots, chopped tomatoes, red wine or water and stock. Stir in the chilli flakes and bay leaf and season with a little salt and lots of ground black pepper. Bring to a simmer on the hob then cover the casserole and transfer to the oven. Cook for 20 minutes.

Take the casserole out of the oven and stir in all the beans. Cover again and return to the oven for a further 15 minutes. Transfer the casserole to the hob and stir in the spring greens or kale. Bring to a simmer and cook for a further 3–5 minutes or until the greens are tender, stirring frequently.

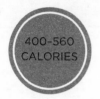

400–560
CALORIES

445

CALORIES
PER SERVING

SERVES 5

**PREP: 15 MINUTES,
PLUS SOAKING
TIME**

COOK: 35 MINUTES

INGREDIENTS

generous pinch of saffron threads

250ml just-boiled water

1 medium onion, finely chopped

1 red pepper, deseeded and cut into roughly
  3cm chunks

1 green pepper, deseeded and cut into
  roughly 3cm chunks

oil, for spraying or brushing

6 boneless, skinless chicken thighs
  (about 500g), trimmed of visible fat
  and cut in half

100g soft cooking chorizo, cut into 5mm
  slices

250g Arborio (risotto) rice

2 garlic cloves, crushed or finely grated

2 tsp hot smoked paprika

100ml dry sherry or extra stock

500ml hot chicken stock (made with
  1 chicken cube)

250g cooked, peeled king prawns, thawed
  if frozen

15g bunch of fresh flat-leaf parsley, leaves
  roughly chopped

flaked sea salt

ground black pepper

oven-baked chicken and prawn paella

A wide-based, fairly shallow casserole works best for this recipe, which is great if you are a bit nervous about cooking rice. I've kept things simple and because the paella is baked in the oven, you should have perfect results every time.

Preheat the oven to 200°C/Fan 180°C/Gas 6. Put the saffron in a measuring jug and add the just-boiled water. Leave to stand for about 10 minutes.

Put the onion and peppers in a shallow flameproof casserole, which holds roughly 2.5 litres. Spray or brush with oil and season with salt and lots of ground black pepper. Fry over a medium heat for 5 minutes, stirring frequently.

Stir in the chicken and chorizo and cook for a further 3 minutes, stirring. Add the rice, garlic, paprika, sherry or stock, plus the saffron and its soaking liquor. Pour over the chicken stock and bring to a simmer. Cover with a lid and cook in the oven for 20 minutes.

Take out of the oven, remove the lid and stir in the prawns and parsley. Cover and return to the oven for a further 5 minutes, or until the prawns are heated through and the rice is tender.

Tip: You can use any sherry; but 100ml of sweet sherry or Madeira contains about 20 calories more than dry sherry.

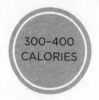

300–400
CALORIES

382
CALORIES
PER SERVING

SERVES: 6

PREP: 20 MINUTES

COOK: 2 HOURS, 40 MINUTES

INGREDIENTS

1 tbsp sunflower oil

1 medium onion, thinly sliced

4 tbsp plain flour

1 tsp flaked sea salt

2 tsp dried mixed herbs

800g lean braising beef (ideally chuck steak), trimmed of hard fat and cut into 3cm cubes

1 bay leaf

500ml bottle real ale

350ml beef stock (made with 1 beef cube)

2 tbsp tomato purée

2 tsp caster sugar

5 medium carrots (each about 100g), peeled and cut into roughly 2cm slices

2 parsnips (each about 150g), peeled, halved lengthways and cut into roughly 2cm chunks

500g medium potatoes (ideally Maris Piper), peeled and cut into roughly 3cm chunks

100g fine green beans, trimmed and halved

ground black pepper

all-in-one beef
and ale stew

The large quantity of vegetables in this stew helps you keep the meat to a minimum. Buy good braising beef – the kind you cut yourself rather than pre-diced – if you can. If you don't want to use beer, add 500ml more beef stock instead. Made with 500ml extra stock, the stew will contain about 357 calories per serving.

Preheat the oven to 180°C/Fan 160°C/Gas 4. Heat the oil in a large flameproof casserole. Fry the onion over a medium-high heat for about 5 minutes until lightly browned, stirring frequently. Remove from the heat.

Put the flour, salt and dried herbs in a large, sturdy freezer bag. Season with lots of freshly ground black pepper. Toss the meat in the flour until coated evenly all over. Tip the meat into the pan with the onions.

Add the bay leaf, ale, stock, tomato purée and sugar. Stir well and bring to the boil. Cover and carefully transfer to the oven. Cook for 1¼ hours. Take the casserole out of the oven, remove the lid and stir in the carrots, parsnips and potatoes. Cover and return to the oven for a further hour, or until the beef is tender.

Stir in the green beans, cover and return to the oven for a further 15 minutes, or until the beans are tender. Adjust the seasoning to taste before serving.

Freeze the cooled stew in a freezer-proof container for up to 2 months. Thaw overnight in the fridge then reheat in the microwave or an ovenproof casserole in a preheated oven at 200°C/Fan 180°C/Gas 6 for 45–60 minutes, stirring after 30 minutes, until piping hot.

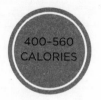

430
CALORIES
PER SERVING

SERVES 5

PREP: 15 MINUTES

COOK: 2¾ HOURS

INGREDIENTS

1 tbsp sunflower oil

2 medium onions, thinly sliced

1kg braising beef (ideally chuck steak), trimmed of hard fat and sinew and cut into roughly 4cm chunks

50g chunk of fresh root ginger, peeled and finely grated

4 garlic cloves, finely grated

1 tsp dried chilli flakes

2 tsp Chinese five spice powder

750ml hot beef stock (made with 1 beef cube)

4 tbsp dark soy sauce

2 tbsp clear honey

2 medium-large carrots, peeled and cut into roughly 1cm diagonal slices

4 tsp cornflour

1 tbsp cold water

250g pouch ready-cooked medium noodles

3 small pak choi, quartered lengthways

ground black pepper

chinese braised beef with noodles

Good-quality braising beef is cooked with Chinese spices, soy sauce and honey until meltingly tender. Cooked noodles and pak choi are added towards the end of the cooking time to make a fabulous one-pot dish. Sprinkle with sliced spring onions or a mixture of finely chopped red chillis and peanuts just before serving. Peanuts are about 150 calories per 25g.

Preheat the oven to 180°C/Fan 160°C/Gas 4. Heat the oil in a large, wide-based flameproof casserole. Fry the onions and beef over a medium-high heat for 10 minutes, or until lightly browned, stirring frequently.

Add the ginger and garlic and cook for a further 2 minutes, stirring. Sprinkle over the chilli and five spice powder and season with lots of ground black pepper. Cook for 1 minute, stirring.

Pour the beef stock, soy sauce and honey into the casserole and stir well. Bring to a simmer, cover and carefully transfer to the oven. Cook for 1½ hours. Add the carrots and cook for 30–45 minutes more or until the beef is very tender.

Take the casserole out of the oven. Increase the oven temperature to 220°C/Fan 200°C/Gas 7. Mix the cornflour with the water until smooth. Stir the noodles and cornflour mixture into the beef, place the pak choi on top, cover and return to the oven for a further 15 minutes or until the pak choi is tender and the noodles are hot.

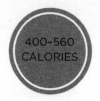

400–560
CALORIES

411
CALORIES
PER SERVING

SERVES 6

PREP: 10 MINUTES

COOK: 2 HOURS

INGREDIENTS

1 tbsp sunflower oil

2 medium onions, finely chopped

2 garlic cloves, crushed

4 tbsp medium curry paste

1.2kg good quality braising beef (ideally
chuck steak), trimmed of hard fat and
sinew and cut into roughly 3cm chunks

1 tsp flaked sea salt

2 x 400g cans chopped tomatoes

200ml beef stock (made with 1 beef cube)

400g potatoes (ideally Maris Piper), peeled
and cut into roughly 4cm chunks

3 medium carrots (about 300g), peeled
and cut into 2cm diagonal slices

150g young spinach leaves

Freeze the cooked and cooled curry in labelled zip-seal bags
or foil containers for up to 2 months. Thaw overnight in the fridge
then reheat in the microwave or a wide-based saucepan over a
medium heat, stirring occasionally until piping hot.

one-pot beef curry

This one-pot beef curry is very easy to make. I save time by using a ready-made medium curry paste – you can choose a mild or hot paste if you prefer. Serve with generous spoonfuls of minted cucumber raita (see page 137).

Preheat the oven to 180°C/Fan 160°C/Gas 4. Heat the oil in a large, flameproof casserole and fry the onion and garlic over a high heat for 1 minute, stirring. Add the curry paste and cook for a few seconds, stirring well.

Add the beef and salt to the pan and cook for 3 minutes, turning the beef regularly until lightly coloured and well coated in the spice paste. Tip the tomatoes into the pan and stir in the beef stock.

Bring the liquid to a simmer, then cover and transfer carefully to the oven. Cook for 1 hour. Take the casserole out of the oven and stir in the potatoes and carrots. Return to the oven for a further hour, or until the beef is beautifully tender and the sauce has thickened.

Place the casserole carefully on the hob and stir in the spinach, just a handful at a time, until softened. Adjust the seasoning to taste and serve with minted cucumber raita (see page 137), if you like.

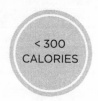

26

CALORIES
PER SERVING

SERVES 6

PREP: 5 MINUTES

INGREDIENTS

½ cucumber

200g fat-free natural yoghurt

2 tsp of mint sauce (from a jar) or 2–3 tbsp
   finely chopped fresh mint

1 tsp caster sugar

flaked sea salt

ground black pepper

easy minted cucumber raita

Yoghurt and mint always go together and are perfect for cooling down a spicy curry. This easy raita uses mint sauce from a jar instead of fresh. I usually keep a jar in my fridge for making quick dips and for adding to lamb casseroles and marinades. Some versions can be quite acidic, so choose carefully. The sugar will help temper any sourness, leaving a lovely minty flavour. Of course, you can also use freshly chopped mint – there is no need to add the sugar then. And quite often, I make without the cucumber too, for an extra quick dip.

Put the cucumber on a board and cut into small chunks. Transfer to a small bowl and season with a little flaked sea salt and some ground black pepper.

Stir in the yoghurt, mint sauce, or fresh mint, and caster sugar, if needed. Leave to stand for 10 minutes before serving to help the flavours develop. This is great served with any of the curries in this book, or the Without The Calories series.

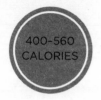

400–560
CALORIES

432
CALORIES
PER SERVING

SERVES 6

PREP: 10 MINUTES, PLUS MARINATING TIME

COOK: 3 HOURS

INGREDIENTS

1kg boned pork shoulder, trimmed of rind
   and fat and cut into 4 large chunks (snip
   off the string and unroll first if necessary)
1 medium red onion, roughly chopped
175ml cold water
12 corn tacos, warmed
1 little gem lettuce, trimmed and finely
   shredded
soured cream or half-fat crème fraiche,
   and lime wedges to serve

For the marinade

3 tbsp chipotle chilli paste (from a jar)
3 tbsp white wine vinegar or cider vinegar
2 tsp dried oregano
1 tsp ground allspice
1 tsp ground cumin
1 tsp flaked sea salt
½ tsp ground cloves
½ tsp ground black pepper

Tip: Heat the tacos on a baking tray in the oven for a few minutes once the pork has been removed.

pibil pulled pork tacos

This isn't a truly authentic Mexican pibil pork recipe, but it's easy to put together with ingredients from the supermarket, and I reckon it tastes pretty close to the original. Soft, succulent and spicy, it's fantastic piled into warm tacos with homemade gently pickled onion (see page 141), shredded lettuce and soured cream (add 31 calories per tablespoon).

Put all the marinade ingredients in a large, sturdy freezer bag and squish them around until well combined. Add the pork and onion and move around in the bag until they are well coated with the marinade. Seal and put in the fridge overnight.

The next day, transfer the pork and its marinade to a small casserole and stir in the cold water. Cover and place in the oven. Set the temperature to 170°C/Fan 150°C/Gas 3 and cook the pork for 3 hours, or until it is so tender that it falls apart when poked with a fork.

Remove the casserole from the oven and shred the meat with two forks. Serve the pulled pork from the casserole or a board with warm corn tacos, shredded lettuce, pickled red onion (see page 141) and soured cream or crème fraiche (but don't forget to add the extra calories), and a squeeze of fresh lime.

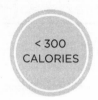

13
CALORIES
PER SERVING

SERVES 6

PREP: 5 MINUTES,
PLUS STANDING

INGREDIENTS

1 medium red onion, peeled

200ml just-boiled water

2 tbsp white wine vinegar or cider vinegar

1 tsp caster sugar

pickled red onion

Lightly pickled red onion is the perfect accompaniment to pulled pork dishes, chilli con carne and spicy grilled or barbecued meats and fish. I use pickled onions like this for tacos and tortillas too. They have a delicious sweet and sour flavour that really lifts a dish, adding not only colour but crunch too.

Put the red onion on a board and carefully cut into thin slices, then break into rings with your fingers. If it helps, you can also cut the onion in half from root to tip and then slice before separating. Throw away the tough root end.

Transfer the sliced onion to a heatproof bowl. Cover with just-boiled water from a kettle and leave to stand for 10 minutes. This will help soften the onion and mellow the flavour.

Once softened, drain the onions well in a sieve over the sink, and return to the bowl. Stir in the vinegar and caster sugar and leave to stand for at least 10 minutes before serving.

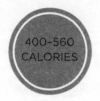

415

CALORIES
PER SERVING

SERVES 6

PREP: 15 MINUTES

COOK: 1½ HOURS

INGREDIENTS

800g lamb neck fillet, trimmed of hard fat and cut into 4cm chunks

4 tsp ras-el-hanout spice mix

1 tsp cumin seeds

2 medium onions, halved and thinly sliced

oil, for spraying or brushing

4 garlic cloves, thinly sliced

750ml hot lamb stock (made with 1 lamb cube)

2 x 400g cans chopped tomatoes

4 tsp harissa paste (preferably rose harissa)

2 tbsp clear honey

400g can chickpeas, drained and rinsed

300g sweet potato, peeled and cut into roughly 3cm chunks

20g bunch of fresh coriander, leaves finely chopped, plus extra to garnish

flaked sea salt

ground black pepper

Flat-freeze the cooked and cooled casserole in two large labelled zip-seal bags for up to 2 months. Thaw overnight in the fridge then reheat in the microwave or a wide-based saucepan, stirring occasionally until piping hot.

moroccan lamb tagine

Lamb tagine always seems to go down well and this simplified version has all the ingredients for a most welcome one pot. There's no need to serve with additional carbohydrates, but you may want to add couscous or rice for anyone not watching their weight. If you don't have ras-el-hanout, mix 2 teaspoons of ground coriander, 2 teaspoons ground cumin, 1 teaspoon ground ginger and 1/4 teaspoon ground cinnamon instead.

Put the lamb in a large, flameproof casserole and season all over with salt and pepper, the ras-el-hanout and cumin seeds. Add the sliced onions and toss together well.

Preheat the oven to 200°C/Fan 180°C/Gas 6. Spray or brush the seasoned lamb and onions with oil and cook over a medium-high heat for about 10 minutes, or until lightly coloured all over, stirring and turning the meat and onions frequently.

Add the garlic and cook for a further 2 minutes, stirring. Pour over the lamb stock, then tip the tomatoes into the pan, add the harissa and honey and bring to a gentle simmer. Cover and cook in the oven for 30 minutes.

Take the casserole out of the oven and stir in the chickpeas and sweet potato. Cover and return to the oven for 45 minutes, or until the lamb is very tender. Sprinkle with chopped coriander and serve with a lightly dressed green salad.

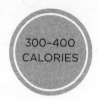

305
CALORIES
PER SERVING

SERVES 4

PREP: 10 MINUTES

COOK: 30–35 MINUTES

INGREDIENTS

20g butter

2 medium leeks (each about 175g), trimmed and cut into roughly 1cm slices

½ small onion, finely chopped

400ml semi-skimmed milk

4 tbsp cornflour

4 tbsp cold water

400g frozen mixed fish for pies

100g frozen cooked, peeled king prawns

flaked sea salt

ground black pepper

For the topping

300g can new potatoes, drained

10g butter

Tip: Packs of frozen mixed fish pieces, containing a mixture of white fish, salmon and smoked fish, are brilliant for this recipe as the fish can be cooked from frozen – often packs of larger prawns can be reheated from frozen too. If you are using thawed or fresh fish, you will need to reduce the cooking time by about 5 minutes.

one-pan fish pie

If you haven't cooked much fish before but fancy trying your hand at a fish pie, this recipe is a great place to start. I've simplified the traditional method and cut the calories to create a dish that's very simple to make and bake.

Preheat the oven to 220°C/Fan 200°C/Gas 7. Melt the butter over a low heat in a small flameproof casserole with a base roughly 23cm in diameter. Add the leeks and onion and cook for 5 minutes or until well softened, stirring frequently.

Pour the milk into the pan and bring to a gentle simmer. Mix the cornflour and water into a smooth paste in a small bowl, then pour into the warm milk. Return to a simmer and cook over a low heat for 2–3 minutes, until the sauce is smooth and very thick, stirring continuously. Season well.

Stir the frozen fish pieces and prawns into the sauce and cook for 2 minutes, stirring gently. Remove from the heat. Coarsely grate the potatoes and scatter over the fish mixture then dot with the butter.

Season with a little ground black pepper and bake uncovered for 20–25 minutes, or until the fish and prawns are hot throughout and the topping is golden.

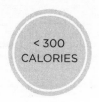

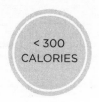

90

CALORIES
PER SERVING

SERVES 5

PREP: 10 MINUTES

COOK: 30 MINUTES

INGREDIENTS

1 tbsp cornflour

150ml red wine

50ml cold water

50g caster sugar

1 cinnamon stick

2 star anise

1 large orange

4 firm but ripe Conference pears

half-fat crème fraiche or single cream,
   to serve

Freeze the cooked and cooled pears in their sauce in a freezer-proof container for up to 1 month. Thaw overnight in the fridge and serve cold or heat gently in the microwave or a wide-based saucepan over a low heat until hot.

mulled pears

Make the most of pears when they are plentiful and poach them in lightly-spiced red wine. You needn't buy expensive wine for this recipe; just use a bottle of cheap plonk and freeze what's left over to liven up a meaty casserole or gravy another day. Add 24 calories per tablespoon for half-fat crème fraiche and 29 for single cream.

Preheat the oven to 190°C/Fan 170°C/Gas 5. Put the cornflour into a medium casserole and stir in 2 tablespoons of the wine until smooth, then add 50ml water, the sugar, cinnamon stick and star anise.

Using a potato peeler, peel the orange in large, wide strips and add them to the pan. Squeeze the orange juice and add to the pan.

Peel the pears and cut them into quarters lengthways. Remove the cores with the tip of a knife. Drop the pear quarters into the wine mixture and place over a medium heat.

Bring the liquid to a simmer, turning the pears a couple of times, then cover the casserole and cook the pears in the oven for 30 minutes, or until just tender. You can test a couple with the tip of a knife.

Serve warm or leave to cool. Place in the fridge until ready to serve (up to 2 days). Serve topped with a little single cream or half-fat crème fraiche.

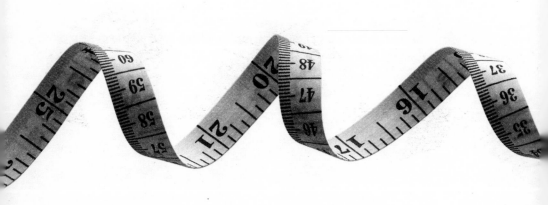

bowl and platter

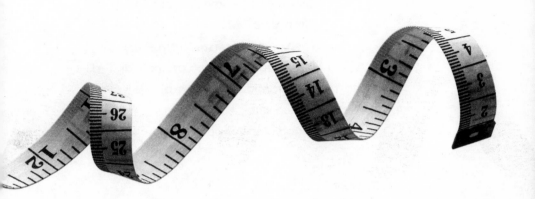

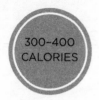

324

CALORIES
PER SERVING

SERVES 6

PREP: 20 MINUTES

COOK: 12 MINUTES

INGREDIENTS

150g uncooked quinoa

875g cold cooked roast chicken (from the chiller cabinet)

400g can red kidney beans, drained and rinsed

200g cherry tomatoes, halved

40g bunch of coriander, leaves roughly chopped

4 spring onions, thinly sliced

1 long red chilli, finely chopped (deseeded first if you like)

1 firm but ripe avocado, stoned, peeled and sliced

For the dressing

fresh juice of 2 limes (about 3 tbsp lime juice)

1 tbsp chipotle paste (from a jar)

1 garlic clove, crushed or finely grated

1 tbsp sunflower or olive oil

fine sea salt

ground black pepper

chicken, quinoa, avocado and chilli salad

The smoky flavour of the dressing for this salad comes from chipotle paste, made from smoked jalapeño peppers. You can find it in the Mexican section of larger supermarkets. Alternatively, add 1 teaspoon of hot smoked paprika to the dressing. Quinoa is a highly nutritious South American seed that can be served in a similar way to rice.

Half fill a medium saucepan with water and bring to the boil. Rinse the quinoa in a fine sieve then add to the water, stir well and simmer for about 12 minutes, or until just tender. It is ready when it begins to shed the c-shaped outer husks.

While the quinoa is cooking, put the chicken on a board and strip off all the meat, discarding the skin and bones. Tear or cut the meat into chunky pieces and put to the side.

Rinse the cooked quinoa in a sieve under cold water, then press hard with a ladle or serving spoon to remove as much of the excess water as possible.

Mix the dressing ingredients in a large bowl. Tip in the quinoa and toss with the dressing ingredients, kidney beans, tomatoes, coriander, spring onions and chilli. Season well with salt and pepper. It's important to make sure that the dressing is mixed well through the salad.

Add the chicken and avocado to the salad and toss everything gently together before serving.

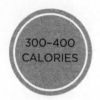

300–400
CALORIES

359
CALORIES
PER SERVING

SERVES 2

PREP: 10 MINUTES

INGREDIENTS

2 cooked boneless, skinless chicken breasts
(200g pack)

2 little gem lettuces, leaves separated,
rinsed and drained

4 spring onions, cut into very fine
matchsticks

⅓ cucumber, cut into very fine matchsticks

1 medium carrot, peeled and cut into very
fine matchsticks

1 small red pepper, deseeded and cut into
very fine matchsticks

fresh coriander leaves, to garnish (optional)

lime wedges, to serve (optional)

For the peanut sauce

2 tbsp crunchy peanut butter

3 tbsp just-boiled water

1 tbsp Thai sweet chilli dipping sauce

1 tbsp dark soy sauce

satay chicken wraps

A brilliant informal supper dish that's easy to prepare and fun to eat. It also makes a great packed lunch, arranged in a lidded container and taken to work.

To make the peanut sauce, put the peanut butter in a small bowl and stir in the just-boiled water until smooth. Add the chilli sauce and soy sauce and mix well.

Cut the chicken breasts into thin slices and put on a large platter. Put the lettuce leaves, spring onions, cucumber, carrot and red pepper in separate piles beside the chicken.

Take the chicken and salad to the table and serve by putting slices of chicken into lettuce leaves and topping with the shredded vegetables and the peanut sauce. Garnish with fresh coriander and serve with extra lime wedges for squeezing over the wraps, if you like.

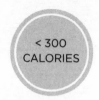

277
CALORIES
PER SERVING

SERVES 2

PREP: 5 MINUTES

COOK: 2 MINUTES

INGREDIENTS

4 small slices of wholegrain bread
  (each slice about 30g)
1 ripe avocado (about 145g)
2 tsp thick balsamic vinegar
ground black pepper

avocado on toast

There is something intensely satisfying about perfectly ripe avocado served on hot toast with a drizzle of balsamic vinegar. It's full of good fats and makes a great light lunch or snack – it beats a cheese sarnie any day.

Toast the bread on both sides and divide the slices between plates. Cut the avocado in half and remove the stone.

Scoop out the flesh and put on a board. Slice the avocado and arrange the slices on the hot toast, mashing them into the toast a little with a knife, then drizzle with the balsamic vinegar. Season with ground black pepper and serve.

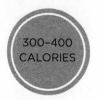

300-400
CALORIES

362

CALORIES
PER SERVING

SERVES 2

PREP: 10 MINUTES

INGREDIENTS

50g bag of rocket leaves

2 firm but ripe nectarines

125g ball of mozzarella, drained

5–6 thin slices prosciutto, Serrano or Parma
ham (about 70g pack)

½ long red chilli, deseeded and finely
chopped

1 tbsp extra virgin olive oil

2 tsp thick balsamic vinegar

ground black pepper

nectarine, prosciutto and mozzarella salad

This is a lovely salad to serve outside on a sunny day. You can use peaches instead of nectarines if you like, and reduced-fat mozzarella if you prefer, but I think the full-fat version has a much better texture and flavour for just 32 calories more per serving.

Scatter the rocket leaves over a serving platter. Take a nectarine and, holding it carefully, cut out slices from top to bottom towards the stone with a small knife, working your way around the whole fruit. You should get 8–10 slices from each nectarine. Discard the stones.

Arrange the nectarine slices on the platter with the rocket leaves and tear the mozzarella on top. Add the prosciutto, torn into wide strips. Sprinkle with the chopped chilli and drizzle with the olive oil and balsamic vinegar. Season with ground black pepper and serve.

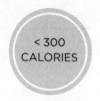

176

CALORIES
PER SERVING

SERVES 6

PREP: 10 MINUTES

INGREDIENTS

1 romaine lettuce, leaves separated

4 medium tomatoes, quartered

½ cucumber, thinly sliced

350g cooked, peeled prawns, thawed if frozen and drained well

pinch of paprika

chopped fresh dill, to garnish (optional)

ground black pepper

lemon wedges, to serve

For the dressing

4 tbsp light mayonnaise

2 tbsp fat-free fromage frais

3 tbsp tomato ketchup

Tip: Use smaller cold-water Atlantic prawns for the best results. If you can't get hold of fat-free fromage frais, use fat-free yoghurt in the dressing instead.

giant prawn cocktail

I love a prawn cocktail and there's no need to exclude it when you are watching your weight, as I've made the dressing with reduced-fat mayonnaise and fromage frais. This one is made in a large dish, but you can serve it in smaller individual dishes if you prefer. One small slice of wholemeal bread spread with 1/4 teaspoon softened butter will add 88 calories to each serving.

To make the dressing, mix the mayonnaise, fromage frais and tomato ketchup in a small bowl.

Arrange the lettuce leaves in a large, wide dish and top with the tomatoes and cucumber. Scatter the prawns on top and spoon over the dressing.

Sprinkle with paprika and ground black pepper. Garnish with fresh dill if you like, and serve immediately with lemon wedges for squeezing and thinly-sliced brown bread.

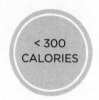

225
CALORIES
PER SERVING

SERVES 2

PREP: 5 MINUTES

INGREDIENTS

300g fat-free Greek yoghurt

1 medium ripe banana

40g dried stoned dates, roughly chopped

15g mixed seeds (such as pumpkin, sesame and sunflower)

2 tsp clear honey (optional)

yoghurt with banana and dates

This yoghurt makes a quick breakfast for busy days. I find the banana and dates sweeten it enough, but you can always add a little honey, too. A teaspoon of honey will increase the calories by 14 per serving.

Divide the yoghurt between two small bowls. Peel and slice the banana and scatter on top. Sprinkle with the dates and seeds and serve drizzled with a little honey, if you like.

Berry yoghurt: Divide 2 x 150g pots of fat-free yoghurt between two bowls. Top with 100g halved, hulled strawberries, 100g raspberries and 50g blueberries. Drizzle with 2 teaspoons clear honey. Serves 2. Calories per serving: 135

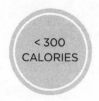

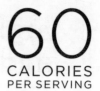

CALORIES
PER SERVING

SERVES 8

PREP: 10 MINUTES

INGREDIENTS

1 small ripe pineapple (about 950g)

1 small cantaloupe melon (about 950g),
   ideally with orange flesh

2 large eating apples (each about 200g)

100g pomegranate seeds

150ml fresh orange juice (from a carton or
   freshly squeezed from 2 oranges)

fat-free Greek yoghurt, to serve (optional)

Tip: Use ready prepared pomegranate seeds from a packet in the chilled fruit section of the supermarket, or buy a large whole pomegranate, remove the seeds yourself and add them and any juice to the salad.

apple, melon, pineapple and pomegranate salad

I like to make this crunchy fruit salad for breakfast and as a snack. It keeps really well in the fridge for around 3 days, which means I can grab a bowl first thing in the morning or whenever I'm feeling a bit peckish. Add 8 calories per tablespoon of fat-free yoghurt.

Place the pineapple on a board and carefully cut off the leaves and skin using a large sharp knife. Pick out any prickly eyes with the tip of a knife. Cut the pineapple into quarters lengthways and remove the central core. Cut the flesh into small, chunky pieces and put in a large bowl.

Cut the melon into six wedges and discard the seeds. Cut carefully between the melon skin and flesh in a long sweeping motion, to separate the flesh from the skin. Cut the flesh into small, chunky pieces. Add to the pineapple.

Cut the apples into quarters and remove the cores. Cut the quarters into roughly 2cm chunky pieces. Add to the other fruit. Scatter the pomegranate seeds over the chopped fruit, stir in the orange juice and toss everything together. Cover and chill for about 1 hour before serving (if you can wait) then divide into dessert dishes or tumblers and top with fat-free Greek yoghurt, if you like.

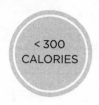

98

CALORIES
PER SERVING

SERVES 5

PREP: 10 MINUTES

INGREDIENTS

1 large ripe mango (about 450g)

2 large eating apples (each about 200g)

150g green seedless grapes, washed
 and drained

150g red seedless grapes, washed and
 drained

150ml fresh orange juice (from a carton
 or freshly squeezed from 2 oranges)

fat-free Greek yoghurt, to serve (optional)

mango, grape and apple salad

A juicy, colourful salad that works well as a pudding, breakfast or snack. The acidity of the orange juice should stop the apples turning brown, so this fruit salad will keep well in the fridge for a couple of days. Add 8 calories per tablespoon of fat-free yoghurt.

Cut the mango in half on either side of the large flat stone. Using a large serving spoon, scoop out the flesh. Cut the mango into small chunks and put in a serving bowl.

Cut the apples into quarters and remove the cores. Cut the quarters into thin slices and add to the mango.

Stir in the grapes, halving any that are particularly large, pour in the orange juice and toss everything together gently. Cover and chill for about 1 hour before serving (if you can wait). Divide into dessert dishes or tumblers and top with fat-free Greek yoghurt, if you like.

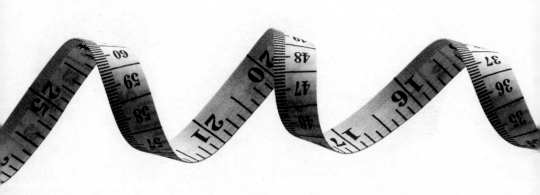

| little pots

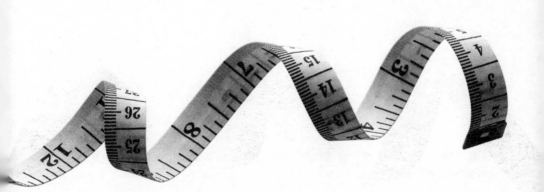

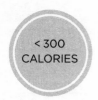

107
CALORIES
PER SERVING

SERVES 6

PREP: 5 MINUTES

COOK: 18 MINUTES

INGREDIENTS

5g softened butter, for greasing

6 medium eggs

4 spring onions, trimmed and thinly sliced

50g sliced smoked salmon

ground black pepper

Tip: These muffins will keep well in the fridge for a day or two in a sealed container.

smoked salmon breakfast muffins

These muffins make a protein-rich breakfast or snack that's easy to transport and can be eaten warm or cold. Serve with a mixed salad for a light lunch if you like, too.

Preheat the oven to 200°C/Fan 180°C/Gas 6. Grease and line a 6-hole muffin tin with squares of baking parchment (about 12cm squares).

Beat the eggs in a jug with a large metal whisk until smooth. Season with black pepper and stir in the sliced spring onions.

Cut the salmon slices into thin strips and divide between the holes of the muffin tin. Pour the egg mixture on top.

Bake the muffins for about 18 minutes, or until the egg is slightly risen and only just set on top – it should still be a little soft, as the egg will continue to cook once the tin has been taken out of the oven. Serve warm or cold.

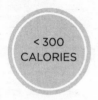

156
CALORIES
PER SERVING

SERVES 6

PREP: 10 MINUTES

INGREDIENTS

4 smoked mackerel fillets (about 225g), skinned
½ small onion
150g quark (fat-free soft cheese)
2 tbsp creamed horseradish sauce
finely grated zest and juice of ½ small lemon
flaked sea salt
ground black pepper
Melba toast and vegetable sticks, to serve

Tips: Ready-made thin Melba toasts go well with this pâté. You'll need to add about 13 calories for each toast and make sure you supplement them with lots of 'free' vegetables (see the list on page 193).

If you can't find quark in your local supermarket, place 200g fat-free fromage frais in a muslin-lined sieve over a bowl and strain it overnight in the fridge.

Freeze the prepared pâté in toughened glass jars or ramekins for up to 1 month. Thaw overnight in the fridge and eat within 24 hours.

smoked mackerel pâté

Smoked mackerel pâté is easy to whizz together and makes a simple starter or snack. It's also great for taking to work, alongside a little bag packed with fresh vegetable sticks. If you don't have a food processor, mash the ingredients together with a sturdy fork.

Flake the mackerel into a food processor. Peel the onion and coarsely grate onto a board. Put the grated onion in one hand and squeeze it hard over the mackerel to release the juice; this will add flavour to the pâté. Discard the onion flesh.

Add the quark, horseradish sauce, lemon zest and juice to the mackerel and season well with a good pinch of salt and plenty of ground black pepper. Blitz all the ingredients together until smooth. Adjust the seasoning to taste and add a little more lemon juice if needed. Spoon the mixture into six small ramekin dishes or little glass Kilner jars and smooth the surface with the back of a teaspoon. Cover and chill.

Take the pâté out of the fridge 20 minutes before serving. Put the ramekins on small plates with Melba toast or vegetable sticks. Eat within 2 days.

400–560
CALORIES

433
CALORIES
PER SERVING

SERVES 2

PREP: 10 MINUTES

INGREDIENTS

200g canned red kidney beans, drained and rinsed

200g canned cannellini beans, drained and rinsed

½ small red onion, thinly sliced

1 medium carrot, peeled and coarsely grated

8 cherry tomatoes, halved

2 romaine lettuce leaves or 1 little gem lettuce, shredded

198g can tuna steak in spring water, drained

flaked sea salt

ground black pepper

For the dressing

1 tsp Dijon mustard

1 tsp caster sugar

1 small garlic clove, crushed

1 tbsp white wine vinegar

4 tbsp olive oil

Tip: Store any unused beans in a covered container in the fridge for up to 2 days. Use for salads, or stir into soups or stews.

tuna and bean layered salad pots

Layered salads are great for packed lunches and picnics. Make sure the dressing stays at the bottom of the dish and only mix the salad just before serving, or it could go soggy. Make it in one large bowl if you are eating at home, or divide between two sturdy containers or pots if you are taking it to work.

To make the dressing, put all the ingredients in a large bowl, add a pinch of salt and some black pepper and whisk with a small metal whisk until slightly thickened.

Add the beans to the bowl and stir in the red onion. (Divide between two lidded containers if you like.) Place the grated carrot, tomatoes and shredded lettuce on top, without stirring.

Flake the tuna out of the can and onto the salad with a fork. Season with pepper. Cover and chill until ready to serve, then lightly toss all the ingredients together.

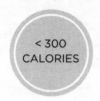

92
CALORIES
PER SERVING

SERVES 4

PREP: 5 MINUTES

INGREDIENTS

400g fat-free Greek yoghurt

3 tbsp lemon curd

100g fresh raspberries

fresh mint leaves and pared lemon zest,
  to decorate (optional)

swirly lemon yoghurt pots

This creamy dessert takes just five minutes to make, but tastes incredibly luxurious – just right when you fancy something sweet, but don't want to wreck your diet.

Put the Greek yoghurt in a bowl and stir until smooth. Add the lemon curd a spoonful at a time and stir it very lightly through the yoghurt. Spoon into glass tumblers or jars and top with fresh raspberries. Decorate with mint leaves and pared lemon zest, if you like.

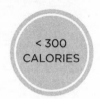

176
CALORIES
PER SERVING

SERVES 4

PREP: 10 MINUTES, PLUS COOLING AND CHILLING TIME

COOK: 5 MINUTES

INGREDIENTS

100g plain dark chocolate (about 50% cocoa solids)

400g fat-free fromage frais

milk chocolate pots

These simple chocolate puddings are made with melted dark chocolate mixed with fromage frais, so they taste light and creamy.

Break 90g of the chocolate into pieces and place in a large heatproof bowl. Set the bowl over a pan of gently simmering water, making sure the bottom of the bowl isn't in contact with the water, until almost melted. (Alternatively, melt in the microwave.) Carefully remove the bowl from the pan and stir the chocolate with a metal spoon until smooth. Leave to cool for about 30 minutes but do not allow to set.

Stir the fromage frais lightly into the melted chocolate. Don't overmix or it will become too runny. Divide the mixture between ramekins or espresso coffee cups. Grate the reserved 10g chocolate on top.

Place on a small tray, cover and chill for at least 1 hour before serving. Eat within 2 days.

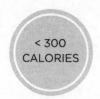

187
CALORIES
PER SERVING

SERVES 4

PREP: 5 MINUTES

INGREDIENTS

3 digestive biscuits

2 medium ripe bananas, sliced

400g fat-free Greek yoghurt

2 tbsp soft light brown sugar

20g tiny fudge pieces (from cake
    decoration section at the supermarket)
    or dairy fudge, cut into small chunks

banoffee yoghurt pots

Banoffee pie is one of my favourite desserts, but is a definite no-no when I'm watching my weight. Here's my low calorie version with all the same elements but given a skinny twist.

Crumble two of the digestive biscuits and divide them between four glasses, dishes or bowls. Top with one of the sliced bananas, spoon over half the yoghurt and sprinkle lightly with half the soft light brown sugar.

Add the remaining banana, yoghurt and brown sugar. Crumble the remaining biscuit on top, sprinkle with tiny fudge pieces and serve.

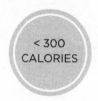

203

CALORIES
PER SERVING

SERVES 8

PREP: 10 MINUTES

COOK: 25 MINUTES

INGREDIENTS

500g frozen mixed summer berries

1 tbsp cornflour

25g caster sugar

low-fat custard or half-fat crème fraiche,
   to serve (optional)

For the topping

25g fridge-cold butter, cut into cubes

20g plain flour

75g corn flakes

summer berry crunch pies

Frozen berries make a quick and convenient low-calorie pudding and are full of vitamins and fibre. You can use them frozen for this recipe or thaw them first if you like, and take 10 minutes off the cooking time. Serve warm with low-fat custard or half-fat crème fraiche, but don't forget to add the extra calories.

Preheat the oven to 200°C/Fan 180°C/Gas 6. Mix the frozen fruit, cornflour and sugar in a large freezer bag, then divide between individual ovenproof dishes and place them on a baking tray.

To make the topping, put the ingredients into the same bag and crush the cornflakes then rub together between your fingertips outside of the bag until they resemble coarse breadcrumbs. This should take 2–3 minutes.

Scatter the topping mixture evenly over the fruit filling. Bake the pies in the centre of the oven for about 25 minutes, or until the fruit filling is hot throughout and the topping is crisp and golden brown.

159
CALORIES
PER SERVING

SERVES 4

PREP: 5 MINUTES

INGREDIENTS

450g fresh ripe strawberries, hulled and
    halved
1 medium ripe banana (roughly 100g peeled
    weight)
3 tbsp blackcurrant cordial
200g fat-free natural yoghurt
25g porridge oats
250ml semi-skimmed milk

Tip: If making ahead, pour the smoothie into lidded containers
and keep in the fridge. You'll need to add extra water or milk, as
the oats will continue to thicken as the smoothie stands.

strawberry, blackcurrant and banana smoothie

This vitamin C-rich smoothie is great for a quick breakfast and can be made the night before and kept in the fridge. Transport it to work in a cool bag and shake well before drinking.

Put the strawberries, banana, blackcurrant cordial, yoghurt and oats in a blender or food processor and blitz to a thick purée.

Add half the milk and blitz until as smooth as possible. Add extra milk, a little at a time, until a drinkable consistency is reached. Pour into tall glasses or jars and serve.

56
CALORIES
PER SERVING

SERVES 6

**PREP: 10 MINUTES,
PLUS FREEZING**

INGREDIENTS

3 ripe medium bananas

100g fat-free natural yoghurt

fresh berries, such as raspberries,

blueberries, strawberries, redcurrants

and black berries, to serve

Tip: You can also use frozen sliced bananas for delicious
smoothies.

low fat banana 'ice cream'

This is a super-quick way to prepare a banana 'ice cream'. It's not an ice cream in the truest sense, but you will be amazed at how delicious and creamy it tastes. You can even make it without the yoghurt if you like. As long as the bananas are fully frozen and you have a sturdy blender or food processor – especially important as you don't want the bowl to crack as you blitz the fruit – you will have great results. It's a great dessert for eating straight away, when it is softly scooped, but can also be frozen in a container. I would still recommend you serve it within 1–2 days though, as it isn't designed for long-term freezing.

Peel the bananas and cut into thick slices. Line a baking tray with greaseproof paper and scatter the banana over a baking tray. Transfer to the freezer and freeze for 4-6 hours, or until solid. Timings will depend on your freezer, but the bananas can be left overnight and up to 2 weeks before using, but I recommend you transfer to a lidded container if freezing for any longer than 24 hours.

Tip into the bowl of a sturdy food processor or blender and add the yoghurt. Blitz until smooth and thickly iced (it's best to use a food processor or blender designed to crush ice).

Serve immediately or scrape into a freezer-proof container, with a rubber spatula and return to the freezer for at least 3–4 hours until firm. Stand at room temperature for a few minutes before serving. Eat just as it is, or serve topped with fresh berries.

a few notes on the recipes

INGREDIENTS

Where possible, choose free-range chicken, meat and eggs. Eggs used in the recipes are medium unless otherwise stated.

All poultry and meat has been trimmed of as much hard or visible fat as possible, although there may be some marbling within the meat. Boneless, skinless chicken breasts weigh about 175g. Fish has been scaled, gutted and pin-boned, and large prawns are deveined. You'll be able to buy most fish and seafood ready prepared but ask your fishmonger if not and they will be happy to help.

PREPARATION

Do as much preparation as possible before you start to cook. Discard any damaged bits, and wipe or wash fresh produce before preparation unless it's going to be peeled.

Onions, garlic and shallots are peeled unless otherwise stated, and vegetables are trimmed. Lemons, limes and oranges should be well washed before the zest is grated. Weigh fresh herbs in a bunch, then trim off the stalks before chopping the leaves. I've used medium-sized vegetables unless stated. As a rule of thumb, a medium-sized onion or potato (such as Maris Piper) weighs about 150g.

All chopped and sliced meat, poultry, fish and vegetable sizes are approximate. Don't worry if your pieces are a bit larger or smaller than indicated, but try to keep roughly to the size so the cooking times are accurate. Even-sized pieces will cook at the same rate, which is especially important for meat and fish.

I love using fresh herbs in my recipes, but you can substitute frozen herbs in most cases. Dried herbs will give a different, more intense flavour, so use them sparingly.

The recipes have been tested using sunflower oil, but you can substitute vegetable, groundnut or mild olive oil. I use dark soy sauce in the test kitchen but it's fine to use light instead – it'll give a milder flavour.

CALORIE COUNTS

Nutritional information does not include the optional serving suggestions. When shopping, you may see calories described as kilocalories on food labels; they are the same thing.

HOW TO FREEZE

Freezing food will save you time and money, and lots of the dishes in this book freeze extremely well. If you don't need all the servings at the same time, freeze the rest for another day. Where there are no instructions for freezing a dish, freezing won't give the best results once reheated.

When freezing food, it's important to cool it rapidly after cooking. Separate what you want to freeze from what you're going to serve and place it in a shallow, freezer-proof container. The shallower the container, the quicker the food will cool (putting it in the freezer while it's still warm will raise the freezer temperature and could affect other foods). Cover loosely, then freeze as soon as it's cool.

If you're freezing a lot of food at once, for example after a bulk cooking session or a big shop, flip the fast freeze button on at least two hours before adding the new dishes and leave it on for twenty-four hours afterwards. This will reduce the temperature of your freezer and help ensure that food is frozen as rapidly as possible.

When freezing food, expel as much air as possible by wrapping it tightly in a freezer bag or foil to help prevent icy patches, freezer burn and discolouration, or flavour transfer between dishes. Liquids expand when frozen, so leave a 4–5cm gap at the top of containers.

If you have a small freezer and need to save space, flat-freeze thick soups, sauces and casseroles in strong zip-seal freezer bags. Fill the bag a third full, then turn it over and flatten it until it is about 1–2cm thick, pressing out as much air as possible and sealing firmly.

Place delicate foods such as breaded chicken or fish fillets and burgers on a tray lined with baking parchment, and freeze in a single layer until solid before placing in containers or freezer bags. This method is called open freezing and helps stop foods sticking together in a block, so you can grab what you need easily.

Label everything clearly, and add the date so you know when to eat it at its best. I aim to use food from the freezer within about four months.

DEFROSTING

Most foods should be defrosted slowly in the fridge for several hours or overnight. For safety's sake, do not thaw dishes at room temperature.

Flat-frozen foods (see page 188) will thaw and begin to reheat at almost the same time. Just rinse the bag under hot water and break the mixture into a wide-based pan. Add a dash of water and warm over a low heat until thawed. Increase the heat, and simmer until piping hot.

Ensure that any perishable foods that have been frozen are thoroughly cooked or reheated before serving.

HOW TO GET THE BEST RESULTS

Measuring with spoons

Spoon measurements are level unless otherwise stated. Use a set of measuring spoons for the best results; they're endlessly useful.

1 tsp (1 teaspoon) = 5ml
1 dsp (1 dessertspoon) = 10ml
1 tbsp (1 tablespoon) = 15ml

A scant measure is just below level and a heaped measure is just above. An Australian tablespoon holds 20ml, so Australian cooks should use 3 level teaspoons instead. See the page 190 for more measurement conversions.

CONVERSION CHARTS

Oven temperature guide

	Electricity °C	Electricity °F	Electricity (fan) °C	Gas Mark
Very cool	110	225	90	1/4
	120	250	100	1/2
Cool	140	275	120	1
	150	300	130	2
Moderate	160	325	140	3
	170	350	150	4
Moderately hot	190	375	170	5
	200	400	180	6
Hot	220	425	200	7
	230	450	210	8
Very hot	240	475	220	9

LIQUID MEASUREMENTS

Metric	Imperial	Australian	US
25ml	1fl oz		
60ml	2fl oz	1/4 cup	1/4 cup
75ml	3fl oz		
100ml	3 1/2fl oz		
120ml	4fl oz	1/2 cup	1/2 cup
150ml	5fl oz		
180ml	6fl oz	3/4 cup	3/4 cup
200ml	7fl oz		
250ml	9fl oz	1 cup	1 cup
300ml	10 1/2fl oz	1 1/4 cups	1 1/4 cups
350ml	12 1/2fl oz	1 1/2 cups	1 1/2 cups
400ml	14fl oz	1 3/4 cups	1 3/4 cups
450ml	16fl oz	2 cups	2 cups
600ml	1 pint	2 1/2 cups	2 1/2 cups
750ml	1 1/4 pints	3 cups	3 cups
900ml	1 1/2 pints	3 1/2 cups	3 1/2 cups
1 litre	1 3/4 pints	1 quart or 4 cups	1 quart or 4 cups
1.2 litres	2 pints		
1.4 litres	2 1/2 pints		
1.5 litres	2 3/4 pints		
1.7 litres	3 pints		
2 litres	3 1/2 pints		

Newport Community
Learning & Libraries

essential extras

Here's my list of suggested 50–150 calorie foods that you can use to supplement the 123 Plan. All calories listed in this list are approximate; a few wayward calories here and there won't make a difference to your allowance. See pages x–xi for more information on essential extras and how they fit into the plan. I've also listed some 'free' vegetable ideas, of which you can eat as much as you like! Make sure your plate is half filled with vegetables or salad, or serve them in a large bowl on the side. Eating more greens will help fill you up and provide lots of extra nutrients in your diet. Your skin will look better and the weight should drop off.

50 CALORIES PER SERVING

30g (about 5) ready-to-eat dried
   apricots
15g (1 tbsp) light mayo
30g (2 tbsp) hummus
40g drained artichoke antipasti
   in oil
60g whole olives
4 fresh apricots
200g fresh blackberries
200g fresh blackcurrants

100g fresh cherries
2 clementines or satsumas
100g fresh figs
½ grapefruit
85g grapes
2 kiwis
100g fresh mango
200g melon
1 medium nectarine
1 medium orange
1 medium peach
1 medium pear
125g fresh pineapple
100g canned pineapple in juice
2 plums
200g papaya
100g pomegranate seeds
200g raspberries
200g strawberries
100g fresh tomato salsa
50g tzatziki
1 level tbsp orange marmalade
1 level tbsp mango chutney
1 level tsp taramasalata
1 level tbsp honey
2cm slice (about 20g) ciabatta
1 x 10g rye crispbread, such as
   Ryvita
50g cooked puy lentils, green lentils
1 x measure (25ml) spirits (light or
   dark, e.g. rum, vodka)
1 tbsp single cream
1 tbsp half-fat crème fraiche

10g Parmesan
30g soft French goat's cheese
25g (1½ tbsp) light soft cheese
150ml orange juice (not from
  concentrate)
100ml regular soy milk
100g low-fat natural yoghurt
50g (about 3 wafer thin slices) of
  ham, turkey or chicken

75 CALORIES PER SERVING

150ml semi-skimmed milk
100g low-fat cottage cheese
25g (small wedge) Camembert
1 tbsp double cream
1 tbsp crème fraiche (full fat)
50g ricotta cheese
¼ 125g ball of fresh mozzarella
¼ average avocado (35g)
50g smoked salmon
1 rasher back bacon, grilled or
  dry-fried
50g cooked, skinless chicken breast
100g cooked jumbo prawns
  (about 9)
1 medium apple
100g blueberries
25g dried mango
2 cream crackers
20g rice cakes (2 or 3)
20g plain breadsticks (about 4)
½ English muffin
1 slice medium white or brown bread
15g shop-bought (not takeaway)
  prawn crackers
1 oatcake
½ 160g tin tuna in brine, drained

40g sun-dried (or sun-blush)
  tomatoes in oil, drained
30g (2 tbsp) raisins
1 medium egg, boiled

100 CALORIES PER SERVING

1 large egg
40g feta cheese
100g plain cottage cheese
50g (2½ tbsp) soured cream
25g blue cheese
100ml fresh custard
25g cooking chorizo
30g ready-to-eat chorizo (about
  5 thin slices)
25g salami (about 5 thin slices)
1 heaped tbsp pesto
45g Parma ham (about 3 slices)
30g smoked mackerel fillet
1 medium banana
1 level tbsp peanut butter
1 tbsp extra virgin olive oil
30g popping corn kernels
20g unsalted plain cashews
20g tortilla chips
25g wasabi peas
20g plain crisps
1 slice of thick cut bread
½ plain bagel
1 x 45g soft white bread roll
½ regular pitta bread
1 slice German style rye bread
1 crumpet
120g baked beans
45g dried couscous
30g dried wholewheat pasta
25g dried soba noodles

30g dried quinoa
125ml wine (white, red, rose)
125ml sparkling wine/Champagne
½ pint lager
½ pint bitter
½ pint dry cider

150 CALORIES PER SERVING

35g Cheddar cheese
100g skinless chicken breast,
    baked or grilled
100g cooked brown rice
115g cooked easy-cook white rice
40g dried basmati rice
1 potato, baked, boiled or mashed
    without fat (195g raw weight)
130g baked sweet potato (about
    ½ large potato)
40g dried rice noodles
50g dried egg noodles
100g cooked pasta
40g porridge oats
50g shop-bought naan bread
    (about ½)
25g unsalted almonds
175ml wine (not sparkling)

'FREE' SAUCES

Brown sauce, in moderation;
    each tbsp is 24 calories
Fish sauce (nam pla)
Ketchup, in moderation; each tbsp
    is 20 calories
Horseradish sauce
Hot sauce (Tabasco)

Mint sauce (not jelly)
Mustard, any variety (English,
    Dijon, wholegrain, American)
Soy sauce
Vinegars (balsamic, white wine,
    malt, etc.)
Worcestershire sauce
Any herbs or spices

'FREE' VEGETABLES

Artichokes, including tinned
    hearts (but not in oil)
Asparagus
Aubergine
Baby sweetcorn
Beans, any green (not baked)
    (French, runner, etc.)
Bean sprouts
Beetroot, fresh, cooked or pickled
Broccoli
Brussels sprouts
Butternut squash
Cabbage, all kinds (Savoy, red,
    white)
Carrots
Cauliflower
Celeriac
Celery
Chicory
Chillies, including pickled jalapeños
Cornichons
Courgettes
Cucumber
Fennel
Garlic
Kale
Leeks

Lemons
Limes
Lettuce and salad greens
    (watercress, baby spinach,
    romaine)
Mangetout
Marrow
Mushrooms
Onions
Peppers

Pickled onions
Radishes
Shallots
Spring onions
Sugar snap peas
Swede
Tomatoes, including tinned (but
    not sun-dried)
Turnips

nutritional information

per serving

quick cheesy chicken and ham   page 3 / serves 4

353 energy (kcal)	1491 energy (kJ)	51.9 protein (g)	22.9 carbohydrate (g)
6.6 fat (g)	2.4 saturated fat (g)	3.6 fibre (g)	1.9 sugars (g)

soda can roast chicken (*without skin)   page 5 / serves 4

539/461* energy (kcal)	2259/1935* energy (kJ)	39.1/43.1* protein (g)	37 / 37 *carb (g)
27.1/16.5* fat (g)	7.2/3.8* satd fat (g)	3.6/3.6* fibre* (g)	2.7/2.7* sugars* (g)

all-in-one roast chicken dinner   page 9 / serves 4

463 energy (kcal)	1952 energy (kJ)	46.9 protein (g)	49.6 carbohydrate (g)
8.9 fat (g)	2.5 saturated fat (g)	11.9 fibre (g)	16.7 sugars (g)

barbecue-style chicken with wedges and corn   page 13 / serves 4

381 energy (kcal)	1609 energy (kJ)	40.3 protein (g)	37.8 carbohydrate (g)
8.7 fat (g)	2.8 saturated fat (g)	3.4 fibre (g)	10.1 sugars (g)

lemony chicken tray bake   page 15 / serves 4

361 energy (kcal)	1525 energy (kJ)	41 protein (g)	37.5 carbohydrate (g)
6.3 fat (g)	1.6 saturated fat (g)	7.5 fibre (g)	14.6 sugars (g)

no-fuss roast lamb   page 17 / serves 6

556 energy (kcal)	2332 energy (kJ)	47.5 protein (g)	45.9 carbohydrate (g)
20.2 fat (g)	6.9 saturated fat (g)	11.7 fibre (g)	14.5 sugars (g)

lamb with spring vegetables and mint   page 21 / serves 2

308 energy (kcal)	1294 energy (kJ)	22.8 protein (g)	35.5 carbohydrate (g)
9.1 fat (g)	3.5 saturated fat (g)	5.3 fibre (g)	12.7 sugars (g)

soy and ginger salmon with noodles   page 23 / serves 4

355 energy (kcal)	1491 energy (kJ)	31.2 protein (g)	24.6 carbohydrate (g)
14.9 fat (g)	2.4 saturated fat (g)	4.2 fibre (g)	14 sugars (g)

warm tuna niçoise   page 25 / serves 2

430 energy (kcal)	1809 energy (kJ)	34.5 protein (g)	41.8 carb (g)
14.9 fat (g)	2.9 sat fat (g)	7.4 fibre (g)	11.4 sugars (g)

vinaigrette   page 27 / serves 2

107 energy (kcal)	442 energy (kJ)	0.2 protein (g)	1.2 carb (g)
11.2 (g)	1.6 sat fat (g)	0.2 fibre (g)	1.2 sugars (g)

one-pan cooked breakfast   page 29 / serves 2

293 energy (kcal)	1218 energy (kJ)	20.7 protein (g)	7.3 carbohydrate (g)
20.2 fat (g)	7.6 saturated fat (g)	1.9 fibre (g)	3.4 sugars (g)

easy apple and blackberry fruit pie   page 31 / serves 6

339 energy (kcal)	1421 energy (kJ)	4.2 protein (g)	41.9 carbohydrate (g)
18.4 fat (g)	5.6 saturated fat (g)	4 fibre (g)	12 sugars (g)

chilli chicken stir-fry with rice   page 35 / serves 4

305 energy (kcal)	1288 energy (kJ)	31.3 protein (g)	35 carbohydrate (g)
5.3 fat (g)	1 saturated fat (g)	3.7 fibre (g)	8.8 sugars (g)

chicken and ham wok lasagne   page 37 / serves 4

467 energy (kcal)	1966 energy (kJ)	56.1 protein (g)	30.4 carbohydrate (g)
11.8 fat (g)	6 saturated fat (g)	2.3 fibre (g)	6.8 sugars (g)

coconut chicken curry   page 39 / serves 4

429 energy (kcal)	1799 energy (kJ)	40.1 protein (g)	29.7 carbohydrate (g)
17.3 fat (g)	7.6 saturated fat (g)	5.1 fibre (g)	9.3 sugars (g)

hoisin meatball stir-fry   page 41 / serves 4

286 energy (kcal)	1195 energy (kJ)	21.3 protein (g)	23.9 carbohydrate (g)
11.9 fat (g)	4.9 saturated fat (g)	5.1 fibre (g)	11.2 sugars (g)

creamy pork, apples and cabbage   page 43 / serves 4

346 energy (kcal)	1459 energy (kJ)	32.1 protein (g)	29.2 carbohydrate (g)
10.6 fat (g)	8.9 saturated fat (g)	7.6 fibre (g)	13.3 sugars (g)

ginger and chilli prawn wraps   page 45 / serves 2

162 energy (kcal)	683 energy (kJ)	19.7 protein (g)	18 carbohydrate (g)
1.6 fat (g)	0.3 saturated fat (g)	4.2 fibre (g)	9.8 sugars (g)

goan fish curry   page 47 / serves 4

286 energy (kcal)	1195 energy (kJ)	25.8 protein (g)	13.3 carbohydrate (g)
14.5 fat (g)	9.4 saturated fat (g)	3.5 fibre (g)	9.4 sugars (g)

paneer and vegetable curry   page 49 / serves 4

367 energy (kcal)	1534 energy (kJ)	19.1 protein (g)	31.5 carbohydrate (g)
18.9 fat (g)	10.8 saturated fat (g)	6.5 fibre (g)	10.2 sugars (g)

vegetable pakoras   page 51 / serves 4

277 energy (kcal)	1141 energy (kJ)	6.8 protein (g)	26.5 carb (g)
14.7 fat (g)	1.7 saturated fat (g)	6.4 fibre (g)	3.8 sugars (g)

minted cucumber yoghurt   page 53 / serves 4

25 energy (kcal)	106 energy (kJ)	2.4 protein (g)	3.8 carb (g)
0.1 fat (g)	0 saturated fat (g)	0.3 fibre (g)	3.4 sugars (g)

leek and potato soup   page 57 / serves 6

140 energy (kcal)	586 energy (kJ)	4 protein (g)	21.3 carbohydrate (g)
4.8 fat (g)	1.8 saturated fat (g)	4.6 fibre (g)	5.7 sugars (g)

carrot, sweet potato and coriander soup   page 59 / serves 6

108 energy (kcal)	455 energy (kJ)	1.8 protein (g)	21.3 carbohydrate (g)
2.4 fat (g)	0.4 saturated fat (g)	5.2 fibre (g)	11.9 sugars (g)

hob-top chicken biryani   page 61 / serves 5

356 energy (kcal)	1487 energy (kJ)	28.2 protein (g)	38.1 carbohydrate (g)
10.2 fat (g)	1.7 saturated fat (g)	6.1 fibre (g)	9.4 sugars (g)

harissa chicken and bulgur pilaf   page 63 / serves 4

328 energy (kcal)	1373 energy (kJ)	27.1 protein (g)	37.9 carbohydrate (g)
8 fat (g)	1.2 saturated fat (g)	3 fibre (g)	1.2 sugars (g)

simple sausage stew   page 65 / serves 4

394 energy (kcal)	1645 energy (kJ)	23.8 protein (g)	23.8 carbohydrate (g)
20.3 fat (g)	6.6 saturated fat (g)	5.1 fibre (g)	12.4 sugars (g)

bolognese pasta pot   page 67 / serves 5

414 energy (kcal)	1744 energy (kJ)	45.7 protein (g)	45.7 carbohydrate (g)
10.6 fat (g)	4.4 saturated fat (g)	2.4 fibre (g)	5.9 sugars (g)

italian fish stew   page 69 / serves 4

365 energy (kcal)	1538 energy (kJ)	27.6 protein (g)	43.9 carbohydrate (g)
6.7 fat (g)	1 saturated fat (g)	4.1 fibre (g)	8.9 sugars (g)

caponata with cannellini beans   page 71 / serves 6

134 energy (kcal)	565 energy (kJ)	23.9 protein (g)	23.9 carb (g)
2.4 fat (g)	0.2 sat fat (g)	4.3 fibre (g)	16.2 sugars (g)

caponata on toast   page 73 / serves 4

378 energy (kcal)	1599 energy (kJ)	14.7 protein (g)	69.4 carb (g)
6.6 fat (g)	0.8 sat fat (g)	7.2 fibre (g)	18.9 sugars (g)

coconut and sweet potato dhal   page 75 / serves 4

378 energy (kcal)	1596 energy (kJ)	61 protein (g)	61 carbohydrate (g)
10 fat (g)	6.1 saturated fat (g)	9.1 fibre (g)	12.2 sugars (g)

fruity tapicoa puddings   page 77 / serves 6

142 energy (kcal)	604 energy (kJ)	28.9 protein (g)	28.9 carbohydrate (g)
1.9 fat (g)	1.2 saturated fat (g)	1.1 fibre (g)	13.1 sugars (g)

lower-fat vanilla ice cream   page 79 / serves 8

130 energy (kcal)	543 energy (kj)	4.7 protein (g)	8.9 carbohydrate (g)
8.7 fat (g)	4.1 saturated fat (g)	0 fibre (g)	8.0 sugars (g)

chicken and vegetable frying pan pie   page 83 / serves 4

377 energy (kcal)	1569 energy (kJ)	32.4 protein (g)	35.3 carbohydrate (g)
10.7 fat (g)	4.5 saturated fat (g)	4.9 fibre (g)	7.7 sugars (g)

italian chicken with mascarpone   page 85 / serves 2

351 energy (kcal)	1474 energy (kJ)	40.7 protein (g)	14.1 carbohydrate (g)
12.5 fat (g)	4.2 saturated fat (g)	2.4 fibre (g)	11.9 sugars (g)

pan-fried pesto chicken   page 87 / serves 2

329 energy (kcal)	1383 energy (kJ)	43.1 protein (g)	18.5 carbohydrate (g)
18.5 fat (g)	15.5 saturated fat (g)	3.8 fibre (g)	15.5 sugars (g)

smoky steak fajitas   page 89 / serves 2

483 energy (kcal)	2035 energy (kJ)	34.9 protein (g)	49.3 carbohydrate (g)
17.6 fat (g)	6.9 saturated fat (g)	6 fibre (g)	11.4 sugars (g)

tortilla chilli pie   page 91 / serves 5

| 352 energy (kcal) | 1476 energy (kJ) | 31 protein (g) | 21.7 carbohydrate (g) |
| 14 fat (g) | 5.7 saturated fat (g) | 6.8 fibre (g) | 7.8 sugars (g) |

moussaka for two   page 93 / serves 2

| 496 energy (kcal) | 2065 energy (kJ) | 30.6 protein (g) | 14.9 carbohydrate (g) |
| 33.5 fat (g) | 17.8 saturated fat (g) | 5.9 fibre (g) | 10.7 sugars (g) |

salmon with puy lentils   page 95 / serves 2

| 498 energy (kcal) | 2083 energy (kJ) | 37.6 protein (g) | 34.7 carbohydrate (g) |
| 21.7 fat (g) | 3.4 saturated fat (g) | 11.2 fibre (g) | 9.8 sugars (g) |

spanish omelette   page 97 / serves 3

| 371 energy (kcal) | 1550 energy (kJ) | 20.9 protein (g) | 25.7 carbohydrate (g) |
| 21.1 fat (g) | 5.9 saturated fat (g) | 4.5 fibre (g) | 9.4 sugars (g) |

warm griddled halloumi salad   page 99 / serves 2

| 499 energy (kcal) | 2074 energy (kJ) | 28.5 protein (g) | 16.7 carbohydrate (g) |
| 35.7 fat (g) | 20.4 saturated fat (g) | 5.4 fibre (g) | 14.1 sugars (g) |

caribbean pineapple   page 101 / serves 4

| 120 energy (kcal) | 507 energy (kJ) | 0.6 protein (g) | 20.2 carb (g) |
| 4.8 fat (g) | 2.1 sat fat (g) | 2 fibre (g) | 20.2 sugars (g) |

baked chicken and mushroom risotto   page 105 / serves 4

| 420 energy (kcal) | 1772 energy (kJ) | 37.2 protein (g) | 47.2 carbohydrate (g) |
| 6.2 fat (g) | 2.9 saturated fat (g) | 2 fibre (g) | 5.4 sugars (g) |

couscous with roasted roots, honey and goat's cheese   page 107 / serves 2

| 416 energy (kcal) | 1751 energy (kJ) | 12.4 protein (g) | 66.9 carbohydrate (g) |
| 11.6 fat (g) | 3.9 saturated fat (g) | 16.1 fibre (g) | 26.6 sugars (g) |

spiced lamb-stuffed courgettes   page 109 / serves 4

| 273 energy (kcal) | 1137 energy (kJ) | 17.3 protein (g) | 24.7 carbohydrate (g) |
| 11.8 fat (g) | 3.7 saturated fat (g) | 1.9 fibre (g) | 6.4 sugars (g) |

salmon and asparagus crustless quiche   page 111 / serves 4

| 254 energy (kcal) | 1058 energy (kJ) | 16.2 protein (g) | 8.4 carbohydrate (g) |
| 17.5 fat (g) | 7.4 saturated fat (g) | 1.6 fibre (g) | 3.0 sugars (g) |

spanish baked fish with chorizo   page 113 / serves 2

416 energy (kcal)	1747 energy (kJ)	42.5 protein (g)	30.6 carbohydrate (g)
14.5 fat (g)	3.7 saturated fat (g)	12.4 fibre (g)	14.3 sugars (g)

chinese rice-stuffed peppers   page 115 / makes 6

104 energy (kcal)	439 energy (kJ)	4.7 protein (g)	17.1 carbohydrate (g)
2.3 fat (g)	0.6 saturated fat (g)	3.9 fibre (g)	8.3 sugars (g)

easy baked apples   page 117 / serves 4

208 energy (kcal)	873 energy (kJ)	2.1 protein (g)	33.3 carbohydrate (g)
8.2 fat (g)	3.5 saturated fat (g)	3.8 fibre (g)	32.9 sugars (g)

nectarine and blueberry muffin cobbler   page 119 / serves 6

251 energy (kcal)	1056 energy (kJ)	6.1 protein (g)	36.9 carbohydrate (g)
9.6 fat (g)	5.1 saturated fat (g)	2.1 fibre (g)	17.4 sugars (g)

quick-mix banana and sultana cake   page 121 / serves 12

173 energy (kcal)	727 energy (kJ)	4.1 protein (g)	25.7 carbohydrate (g)
6.7 fat (g)	1.1 saturated fat (g)	1.3 fibre (g)	9.7 sugars (g)

tarragon chicken   page 125 / serves 4

321 energy (kcal)	1342 energy (kJ)	28.2 protein (g)	19.7 carbohydrate (g)
13 fat (g)	7 saturated fat (g)	5.1 fibre (g)	7.6 sugars (g)

simple cassoulet   page 127 / serves 5

480 energy (kcal)	2008 energy (kJ)	42.7 protein (g)	28.6 carbohydrate (g)
20 fat (g)	6.8 saturated fat (g)	7.7 fibre (g)	10.7 sugars (g)

oven-baked chicken and prawn paella   page 129 / serves 5

445 energy (kcal)	1875 energy (kJ)	40.3 protein (g)	45.7 carbohydrate (g)
8.9 fat (g)	3 saturated fat (g)	2.3 fibre (g)	5.2 sugars (g)

all-in-one beef and ale stew   page 131 / serves 6

382 energy (kcal)	1606 energy (kJ)	32.1 protein (g)	39.2 carbohydrate (g)
10.2 fat (g)	3.4 saturated fat (g)	8.6 fibre (g)	15.7 sugars (g)

chinese braised beef with noodles   page 133 / serves 5

430 energy (kcal)	1812 energy (kJ)	43.7 protein (g)	33.9 carbohydrate (g)
13.3 fat (g)	4.7 saturated fat (g)	4.7 fibre (g)	14.5 sugars (g)

one-pot beef curry page 135 / serves 6

411 energy (kcal)	1724 energy (kJ)	44.7 protein (g)	25.5 carb (g)
15 fat (g)	4.9 saturated fat (g)	5.7 fibre (g)	11.7 sugars (g)

minted cucumber raita page 137 / serves 6

26 energy (kcal)	108 energy (kJ)	2.1 protein (g)	4.3 carb (g)
0.1 fat (g)	0 saturated fat (g)	0.3 fibre (g)	4.2 sugars (g)

pibil pulled pork tacos page 139 / serves 6

432 energy (kcal)	1803 energy (kJ)	34.5 protein (g)	18.2 carb (g)
24.2 fat (g)	6.2 sat fat (g)	1.9 fibre (g)	2.4 sugars (g)

pickled red onion page 141 / serves 6

13 energy (kcal)	53 energy (kJ)	0.3 protein (g)	2.7 carb (g)
0 fat (g)	0 sat fat (g)	0.5 fibre (g)	2.1 sugars (g)

moroccan lamb tagine page 143 / serves 6

415 energy (kcal)	1737 energy (kJ)	30 protein (g)	29.6 carbohydrate (g)
20.4 fat (g)	8.4 saturated fat (g)	6 fibre (g)	13.5 sugars (g)

one-pan fish pie page 145 / serves 4

305 energy (kcal)	1285 energy (kJ)	29.2 protein (g)	22 carbohydrate (g)
11.8 fat (g)	6 saturated fat (g)	3.2 fibre (g)	7.4 sugars (g)

mulled pears page 147 / serves 5

90 energy (kcal)	384 energy (kJ)	0.4 protein (g)	19 carbohydrate (g)
1 fat (g)	0 saturated fat (g)	1.5 fibre (g)	17.8 sugars (g)

chicken, quinoa, avocado and chilli salad page 151 / serves 6

324 energy (kcal)	1360 energy (kJ)	27.8 protein (g)	23.2 carbohydrate (g)
13.9 fat (g)	3 saturated fat (g)	5.1 fibre (g)	4.7 sugars (g)

satay chicken wraps page 153 / serves 2

359 energy (kcal)	1504 energy (kJ)	37.8 protein (g)	18.8 carbohydrate (g)
15.2 fat (g)	3.8 saturated fat (g)	5.4 fibre (g)	13 sugars (g)

avocado on toast page 155 / serves 2

277 energy (kcal)	1159 energy (kJ)	7.1 protein (g)	28.7 carbohydrate (g)
15.6 fat (g)	3.2 saturated fat (g)	7.5 fibre (g)	3.9 sugars (g)

nectarine, prosciutto and mozzarella salad   page 157 / serves 2

362 energy (kcal)	1512 energy (kJ)	23.6 protein (g)	16.2 carbohydrate (g)
22.9 fat (g)	10.9 saturated fat (g)	2.8 fibre (g)	16 sugars (g)

giant prawn cocktail   page 159 / serves 4

176 energy (kcal)	738 energy (kJ)	22.2 protein (g)	9.3 carbohydrate (g)
5.7 fat (g)	1 saturated fat (g)	2.7 fibre (g)	8.5 sugars (g)

yoghurt with banana and dates (*berry yoghurt)   page 161 / serves 2

225/135* energy (kcal)	974/576* energy (kJ)	18.4/9.4* protein (g)	32.4/24.2* carb (g)
3.7/0.6* fat (g)	0.6/0.2* sat fat (g)	2.4/2.4* fibre (g)	30.1/22.8* sugars (g)

apple, melon, pineapple and pomegranate salad   page 163 / serves 8

60 energy (kcal)	258 energy (kJ)	1 protein (g)	14.5 carbohydrate (g)
0.2 fat (g)	0 saturated fat (g)	3 fibre (g)	14.5 sugars (g)

mango, grape and apple salad   page 165 / serves 5

98 energy (kcal)	418 energy (kJ)	1 protein (g)	24.6 carbohydrate (g)
0.2 fat (g)	0 saturated fat (g)	3.5 fibre (g)	24.5 sugars (g)

smoked salmon breakfast muffins   page 169 / serves 6

107 energy (kcal)	446 energy (kJ)	9.5 protein (g)	0.2 carbohydrate (g)
7.6 fat (g)	2.3 saturated fat (g)	0.1 fibre (g)	0.2 sugars (g)

smoked mackerel pâté   page 171 / serves 6

156 energy (kcal)	645 energy (kJ)	10.1 protein (g)	2.4 carbohydrate (g)
11.7 fat (g)	2.3 saturated fat (g)	0.1 fibre (g)	2 sugars (g)

tuna and bean layered salad pots   page 173 / serves 2

433 energy (kcal)	1806 energy (kJ)	27 protein (g)	28.5 carb (g)
24 fat (g)	3.5 saturated fat (g)	8 fibre (g)	11.2 sugars (g)

swirly lemon yoghurt pots   page 175 / serves 4

92 energy (kcal)	405 energy (kJ)	10.7 protein (g)	12.2 carbohydrate (g)
0.6 fat (g)	0.2 saturated fat (g)	0.8 fibre (g)	9.7 sugars (g)

milk chocolate pots   page 177 / serves 4

176 energy (kcal)	742 energy (kJ)	8.9 protein (g)	20.5 carbohydrate (g)
7.1 fat (g)	4.3 saturated fat (g)	0.8 fibre (g)	20.1 sugars (g)

banoffee yoghurt pots	page 179 / serves 4		
187 energy (kcal)	805 energy (kJ)	11.7 protein (g)	31.4 carbohydrate (g)
2.8 fat (g)	1.4 saturated fat (g)	0.7 fibre (g)	24.9 sugars (g)
summer berry crunch pies	page 181 / serves 4		
203 energy (kcal)	855 energy (kJ)	3.2 protein (g)	37.1 carbohydrate (g)
5.6 fat (g)	3.4 saturated fat (g)	4 fibre (g)	16.1 sugars (g)
strawberry, blackcurrant and banana smoothie	page 183 / serves 4		
159 energy (kcal)	672 energy (kJ)	6.7 protein (g)	30.2 carbohydrate (g)
1.9 fat (g)	0.8 saturated fat (g)	2.6 fibre (g)	25.6 sugars (g)
banana 'ice cream'	page 185 / serves 4		
56 energy (kcal)	240 energy (kJ)	1.5 protein (g)	13 carb (g)
0.2 fat (g)	0.1 sat fat (g)	0.7 fibre (g)	11.8 sugars (g)

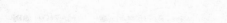

index

acknowledgements

Firstly, huge thanks to everyone who enjoys my recipes and the way I cook. You have given me such fantastic feedback; I hope you like these dishes just as much.

An enormous thank you to John, Jess and Emily for tasting and appraising over 500 new recipes in the past 18 months!

I'm truly grateful to the very talented photographer Cristian Barnett for wonderful photographs that really make my food come to life. And the brilliant Claire Bignell for her superb creative skills, selecting the perfect props and helping make the recipes look both beautiful and achievable. Massive thanks to Lauren Brignell for all her invaluable nutritional support and the hundreds of recipes she has analysed over the past few months. Also, thanks to Rebecca Roberts for carefully testing recipes and assisting on shoot days. Not forgetting Annabel Wray, Annie Simpson and Charlotte Page for their hard work in the test kitchen.

At Orion, I would like to thank Amanda Harris for believing in this project right from the beginning and for trusting me to get on and develop the series. Also thank you to Jillian Young, my fantastic editor, for her guidance and professionalism and Helen Ewing for her design support.

I'm also grateful to my agent, Zoe King, at The Blair Partnership, for her constant encouragement and enthusiasm.

And a final heartfelt thank you to my family and my friends for their fantastic support.

about the author

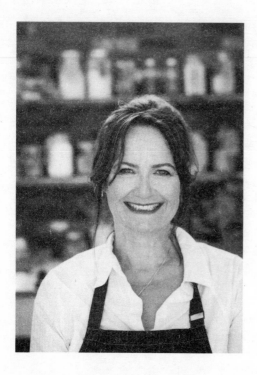

Justine Pattison is one of the UK's favourite healthy eating
cookbook authors. To date, her recipes have featured in books
totalling over 5 million sales. She contributes to the BBC Food
website, consults for various television programmes and
appears regularly on ITV This Morning. She co-authored *The
Fast 800 Recipe Book* and is also the author of *Fill Your
Freezer* and the *Without the Calories* series, which has sold
over 200,000 copies. Join her online community at
justinepattison.com.